MW01615396

The Fundamentals
of Homotoxicology

Diagnosis and Therapy

of Homotoxicoses

The Fundamentals of Homotoxicology

Diagnosis and Therapy of Homotoxicoses

Gabriele Herzberger

Prof. Dr. Hartmut Heine · Gisela King

Erich Reinhart · Bruno Van Brandt

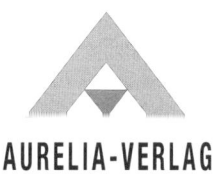

AURELIA-VERLAG

Gabriele Herzberger, M.D.

© 2001 by Aurelia-Verlag GmbH
Postfach 115, D-76481 Baden-Baden
Dr.-Reckeweg-Straße 2-4, D-76532 Baden-Baden

Typesetting and printing by
Franz W. Wesel Druckerei und Verlag GmbH & Co. KG,
Baden-Baden
Printed in Germany

1st English edition 2001
ISBN 3-922907-82-2
70002670 8/2001 WE

Table of Contents

1. Medical Classification Systems

As a result of massive increases in environmental loading and many other consequences of modern civilization, today's medicine is confronted with a series of grave problems. All our scientific and technological progress, our wealth of detailed medical knowledge, and our extremely detail-oriented medical technology have failed to produce decisive breakthroughs in human health.

What is the current situation?

The field of medicine has experienced a paradigm shift from formerly devastating plagues and infectious diseases to chronic and degenerative disorders (diseases of civilization). In addition, there have been major increases in allergic and pseudo-allergic hypersensitivity and intolerance reactions. Although treatments for acute illnesses achieve very high rates of success, chronic diseases pose increasing problems. (The proportion of chronic to acute diseases was approximately 1:1 in 1900; today it is 9:1) The effects of a degraded environment and the aging of the population have contributed to this shift, which suggests that the human body has reached its limits of tolerance and is now being subjected to ongoing excessive demands that irritate and weaken the immune system. In the long run, exclusively symptomatic treatment of the resulting illnesses and the targeted use of higher doses of allopathic medications cannot produce satisfactory results. Understandably, many practitioners now acknowledge the need to factor in endogenous systems and seek holistically oriented forms of therapy.

To what extent can the homotoxicology of Hans-Heinrich Reckeweg (1905-1985) meet such demands and decisively strengthen, support, relieve, and protect our self-healing mechanisms? To explain homotoxicology, we must first clarify the principles underlying conventional methods and the differences and similarities between these two schools of medical thought.

1.1 Historical Context

Until the beginning of the scientific era approximately 100 years ago, Western medicine was based on Hippocratic humoral pathology. Hippocrates postulated that "Health depends first and foremost on the composition of the body's fluids." He called disturbances in these fluids (the disorders we now call metabolic diseases) "dyscrasia." Modern clinical medicine, however, is based on Virchow's theory of cellular pathology. Rudolf Virchow (1821-1902), a pathologist whose theory reduced illnesses to changes in individual cells, held that diseases were triggered by specific, localized disorders rather than by changes in the entire organism. In contrast to the static nature of cellular pathology, humoral pathology recognizes the dynamics involved in all manifestations of life.

Hans Eppinger (1879-1946) was the first to recognize the importance of the system of extracellular fluids that allows blood and lymph to nourish cells and remove the waste products of metabolism. On the basis of Eppinger's work, the pathologist and histologist Alfred Pischinger (1899-1983) studied the functions of connective tissue (mesenchyme), recognizing it as the organic substrate of the living organism's basic regulatory processes. In addition to being the sounding board for all stimuli that reach the body's periphery along neurohumoral or hemohumoral pathways, extracellular fluid also serves the exchange of oxygen, water, and electrolytes, the regulation of acid-base balance, and the activities of the unspecific defense system (Figure 1). The system of extracellular matrix (ground substance) always responds holistically, as an anatomical and functional unity. All nutrients and medications pass through it, and we have learned to measure its responses.

Pischinger and his colleagues made it their life's work to establish a theoretical basis for holistic medicine and to rediscover the significance of humoral pathology. Thus, Pischinger's model provides important prerequisites for a new approach to holistic medicine in that it is oriented toward the totality. This work is continued by the German anatomist Heine, head of the Institute of Antihomotoxic Medicine and Ground Regulation Research in Baden-Baden (Germany).

Pischinger's theories and the results of his research have been largely corroborated by work in the fields of colloidal chemistry,

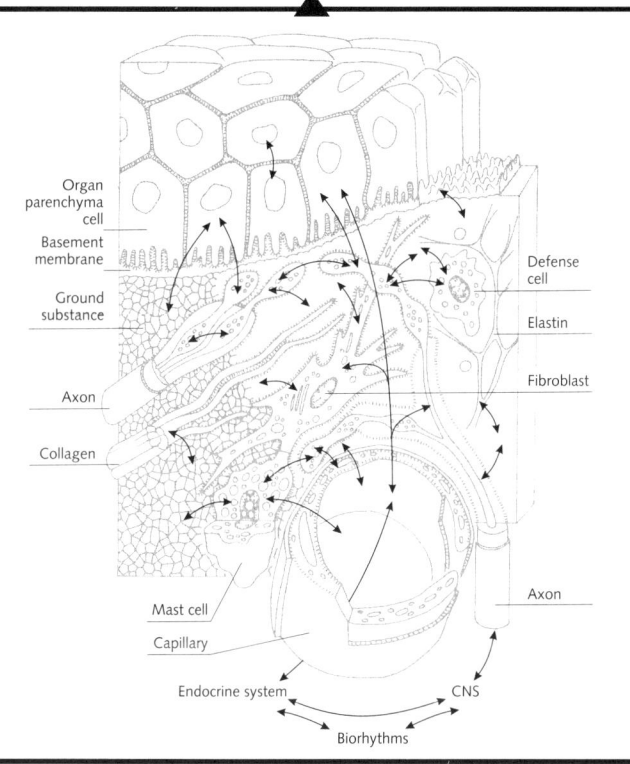

Organ parenchyma cell
Basement membrane
Ground substance
Axon
Collagen
Mast cell
Capillary
Endocrine system
Biorhythms
Defense cell
Elastin
Fibroblast
Axon
CNS

Fig. 1: Scheme of ground regulation according to Heine

molecular biology, enzymology, allergology, and immune research.

1.2 An Overview of Medical Methodologies

The classification systems of conventional medicine categorize illnesses either by type (acute or chronic; inflammatory or degenerative) or according to the organs affected. For lack of suitable categories, syndromes are frequently given the names of their discoverers (Table 1).

By diseased organ	By type of illness	By name of discoverer
Cardiac	Acute	Roemheld's syndrome
Pulmonary	Chronic	Parkinson's disease
Gastric	Inflammatory	Alzheimer's disease
Kidney	Degenerative	Raynaud's disease

Tab. 1: Classification of diseases (14)

In conventional medicine, which sees symptoms as the end results of an unbroken, traceable pathogenetic chain, pathology and anatomy tend to be organ-related.

Tables 2 and 3 describe the types of medications traditionally used in medicine.

Conventional medicine essentially applies scientific methodology to the diagnostic process. Typically, similar symptoms are observed in different patients, a coherent picture of the illness is developed, and a syndrome or symptom complex is then described. Ultimately, this syndrome is divorced from any individual patient and becomes the standard for therapy. The illness is reduced to measurable parameters, and the patient plays a passive role. The goal of therapy is to eliminate symptoms; once this is achieved, the patient is considered cured. Within limits, adverse effects are expected and tolerated.

Before scientific methods of examination and treatment existed, medicine obeyed holistic laws, attempting to stimulate endogenous defense forces and eliminate noxae to reestablish the function

Substitution	Iron replacement for iron-deficiency anemia insulin for insulin-dependent diabetes
Suppression	Cortisone for allergies
Compensation	Spasmolytics, sedatives
Allergens	Desensitization using minimal doses
Homeopathic/antihomotoxic remedies	Stimulation of self-healing processes
Placebos	Their effects can substitute for those of compensatory medication but never those of substitutive or suppressive medication.

Tab. 2: Types of medications, adapted from Spitzy (modified by John) (17, 33)

Artificial Therapy Direct, easily quantifiable pharma- cological effects	• Substitution • Elimination (suppression, e.g., of pathogens or bodily func- tions)
Natural Therapy Secondary effects that are difficult to quantify (therapeutic efficacy)	• Manipulation of processes (compensation)

Tab. 3: Artificial and natural therapy according to Virchow, as modified by John (17, 38)

of the entity consisting of body, mind, and spirit. In the last 150 years, however, analytical thinking and methodology have led the field of medicine out of this empirical phase and into the scientific stage. On the one hand, this shift has produced impressive results; on the other, analytical thinking has led to a dead end in that its focus on single causes has proved incapable of explaining complex and dynamic disease processes.

Of necessity, the older, holistic view of medicine lost ground when confronted with increasingly refined scientific methods and detailed, differentiated knowledge. The resulting fragmentation of medicine into specialties has led to advances in surgery and organ transplantation and in substitution therapy for metabolic disorders, to list only a few examples. The opposite development can be observed, however, with regard to the treatment of chronic illnesses such as vegetative regulatory disorders, cancer, rheumatic diseases, and multiple sclerosis, in which multifactorial origins largely eliminate the possibility of treatment based on linear, causal reasoning. Thinking in terms of single causes provides at best a partial understanding of specialized processes. Thus, to find effective solutions to the problems of treating chronic illnesses, we have had to increase our understanding of dynamic interactions in biological systems, which – as information from the fields of cybernetics and open-system thermodynamics clearly demonstrates – are by no means linear but highly interconnected and subject to a fluid state of biological balance, or "steady state," because they constantly exchange energy and matter with their surroundings (Bertalanffy).

1.3 The Fundamentals of Regulatory Medicine

Pischinger's fundamental research, continued by Heine, described the matrix regulation system as a physiological system of capillaries, connective tissue cells, and autonomic nerve endings all functioning within the extracellular fluid (now called extracellular matrix or ground substance) (Figure 1). This concept supports attempts to update holistic perspectives and serves as a bridge between the past, present, and future of medicine.

Regulatory medicine (from the Latin *regulare*, to bring into order) makes use of pattern recognition ("manifestations of life") as it attempts to understand complex interrelationships and implement therapies that bring order to them. Consequently, acute symptoms constitute only one part of anamnestic and diagnostic analysis in regulatory medicine. The acute episode remains in an individual context and can be treated holistically according to the regulatory principle ("helping the body help itself") of complementary or biological medicine. In contrast, conventional medicine works on the principle of "finding the key that fits the keyhole," attempting first to discover direct, objective, cause-and-effect relationships independent of the individual (ideally, on the molecular level) and then to quantitatively eliminate the molecules responsible for the acute situation.

Although conventional medical therapy (e.g., corticoids) may indeed achieve rapid results, long-term implementation often results in severe adverse effects. A recent study published in *The Journal of the American Medical Association* (Lazarone I et al. Incidence of adverse drug reactions in hospitalized patients. A meta-analysis of prospective studies. JAMA 1998; 279:1200–5) concluded that the more specific the relationship between the therapy and the disorder (for example, using a specific antibody to influence a specific receptor), the more serious the long-term adverse effects are likely to be. With the exception of the "lightning reaction" in Huneke's neural therapy, the effects of regulatory procedures are generally less rapid, but they tend to be long-lasting. In many cases, therefore, combining the two schools of therapy is appropriate; that is, while the methods of one or the other may be justified in specific instances, they are often mutually dependent. The use of homeopathic and antihomotoxic remedies makes eminent sense from the perspective of regulatory medicine if both the fundamental biological law or Arndt-Schulz law (which states that weak stimuli induce regulatory processes) and the complexity of the underlying disorders are taken into account. Potentization increases the energy of the plant, animal, or mineral extracts used, thus allowing certain chemical compounds to form more readily and others to be more easily dissolved.

The system of matrix regulation, as explained below, constitutes the scientific basis of regulatory medicine.

1.3.1 The Concept of Regulation

The cybernetic concept of "regulation through control" is exemplified in the control loop with its variables (sensing element, actual value, desired value, control element), which are interconnected through feedback loops. Originally, *regulatio* (Latin) did not mean approaching a norm in any technical sense but rather an individual's learning about and observing a *nomos*, an ethical position permitting an outlook on life in harmony with nature and one's fellow human beings. Such a position is associated with concern for maintaining the unity of body, mind, and spirit – that is, individual health.

It is impossible to observe the function of a single isolated feedback loop in a clinical setting, but it is possible to observe regulatory systems such as reflex pathways or the functional link among hypothalamus, hypophysis, and adrenals (the so-called stress response pathway). A regulatory system always presupposes a system of interrelated desired values. The goal is to maintain homeostasis (a state of approximate physiological balance) under fluctuating environmental conditions. Homeostasis represents a multidimensional desired value around which an actual value oscillates as a permissible difference (tolerance), allowing the system to correct disturbance-triggered deviations with little loss of energy. An open energy system requires inputs of suitable energy (in the form of nourishment or appropriate therapy, for example) and elimination of expended energy to maintain or restore a labile state of order by means of biorhythms. To survive, therefore, a system must either be in resonance with itself and its environment or must be able to re-create this state continually. Such concepts form the theoretical basis for diagnostic acupuncture tests (such as electroacupuncture), bioresonance procedures, and kinesiology. As soon as an organism (which can be seen as an oscillating circuit from the electromagnetic perspective) is inserted into the circuit of an electromagnetic measuring device, it begins to function like a radio receiver/transmitter. In acupuncture, a metal honeycomb-like device with multiple holes into which test vials can be inserted represents the "antenna" that is needed to adjust the frequency. Inserting test substances into this device adjusts the receiver to normal resonance. The appropriate substance can then be administered in the form of a therapeutic agent ("vegetative antenna"). Kinesiological testing of medications works similarly. Bioresonance procedures attempt to cancel out pathological oscillations by feeding in appropriate counteroscillations.

The circadian rhythm is especially significant in this context. Its diurnal phase is predominantly sympathicotonic and anabolic, its nocturnal phase vagotonic and anabolic. Individual normalcy falls within the range of acceptable tolerance of these two polar neurovegetative systems. Under normal circumstances, any regulatory disorder in the organism is eliminated by a sympathicotonic alarm response (shock phase) and a vagotonic countershock phase, after which the fundamental rhythm reasserts itself (usually in a 7-day cycle) (Figure 3).

A lasting, one-sided shift in this balance leads to dysregulation. In the clinical symptom complex (syndrome X) that combines insulin resistance, glucose intolerance, hyperinsulinemia, elevated very-low-density lipoprotein levels, decreased high-density lipoprotein cholesterol levels, and hypertension, for example, the dysregulation is supported by sympathicotonia (rigidification of matrix regulation in the shock phase) while in gynecological disorders it is mostly supported by vagotonia (rigidification in the countershock phase) (Figure 2).

The sympathetic nervous system, which controls episodes of pain and an individual's degree of wakefulness, is centrally dependent on its anabolic partner, the vagus nerve (parasympathetic nervous system). The exudative shock phase may also alternate with the proliferative countershock phase, as in rheumatoid arthritis. Completely irregular shifts in regulation occur in patients with tumors. The phase of a regulatory disorder can be determined by measuring electrolyte levels in a whole blood sample (Figure 2).

Thus one universal principle of regulatory medicine is: When the relationship between catabolic and anabolic regulators is not

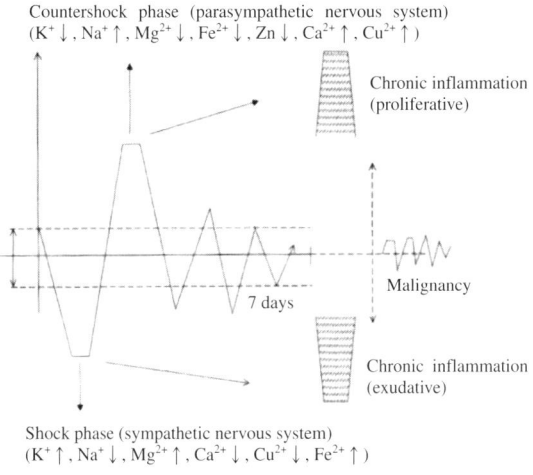

Countershock phase (parasympathetic nervous system)
($K^+ \downarrow$, $Na^+ \uparrow$, $Mg^{2+} \downarrow$, $Fe^{2+} \downarrow$, $Zn \downarrow$, $Ca^{2+} \uparrow$, $Cu^{2+} \uparrow$)

Chronic inflammation (proliferative)

Malignancy

7 days

Chronic inflammation (exudative)

Shock phase (sympathetic nervous system)
($K^+ \uparrow$, $Na^+ \downarrow$, $Mg^{2+} \uparrow$, $Ca^{2+} \downarrow$, $Cu^{2+} \downarrow$, $Fe^{2+} \uparrow$)

Fig. 2: Stimulus-response behavior in the matrix regulation system. Vagotonic counterregulation follows the sympathicotonic shock response, accompanied by corresponding changes in blood electrolyte levels. Matrix regulation can become stuck in either the shock or the countershock phase (chronic illnesses); irregular oscillation (so-called "regulation rigidity") is typical of malignancies.

optimal, regulatory disorders develop. Such disorders become chronic when the regulator irreversibly alters the desired value, leading to a change in the entire feedback relationship (mobilization of the autonomic nervous system). The transition from physiological tolerance to a stable but false desired value is reflected in a maladaptation syndrome that involves increases in anaerobic metabolism, carbonic acid, and latent tissue acidosis (due to increases in lactic acid and free radicals, among other factors). The result is a generalized proinflammatory situation that leads to a vicious circle and chronic illness. In principle, all detoxifying and deblocking measures (such as fasting, dietary changes, orthomolecular medicine, and meditative practices) help control latent acidosis. The transition from tolerance to mobilization of the autonomic nervous system constitutes a *biological division* beyond which a disease process, having invariably passed through an inflammation phase, becomes first chronic and then degenerative.

Medical Classification Systems

1.3.2 The Ground (Matrix) Regulation System

Matrix regulation research has shown that the functions of cells depend to a significant extent on the composition of the extracellular milieu or matrix that surrounds them (Figure 1). Organ cells are not in direct contact with terminal vessels or nerve endings, and even myoneural or neural synapses have gaps filled with polymeric sugars. Any influence that reaches cells and cell parenchymas must pass through the matrix, which regulatory medicine sees as playing the central role. (In contrast, conventional medicine casts the individual cell and its genome in this role.) The matrix is constantly adapting to specific situations, and exogenous and endogenous influences determine its age-appropriate condition ("steady state").

For the most part, the structure of the extracellular matrix is known. The space between terminal vessels and organ cells is occupied by a molecular sieve of highly polymerized glycoproteins and polysaccharides (proteoglycans and glycosaminoglycans; PG/GAGs) intertwined with structural proteins (collagen, elastin) and connective glycoproteins (e.g., fibronectin). As a result of the piezoelectric and pyroelectric properties of collagen, all mechanical and thermal influences cause the formation of electromagnetic fields that activate cells and nerves when fed into the matrix. One explanation for the value of mechanical exercises (walking, running, massage) is that the matrix consumes influxes of mechanical energy by increasing viscoelectricity. PG/GAGs bind water in structured, liquid-crystalline forms, creating a rapid system for the transmission of information (e.g., pH changes). By increasing the temperature and thus also the proportion of fluid, a fever can eliminate faulty information.

In addition to binding water, PG/GAGs are capable of ion exchange and therefore ensure equal levels of ions, electrolytes, and osmotic pressure in the tissues. PGs are capable of forming tunnel structures in the nanometer range (~100 nm). These tunnels transport lipophilic substances in their interiors and hydrophilic substances along their outer walls (guest-host complexing).

Substances are transported by a rapid assembly-disassembly process of the tunnels through the matrix along pH gradients, convection currents, concentration gradients, etc. Since the transport of substances to and from the cells depends on this process,

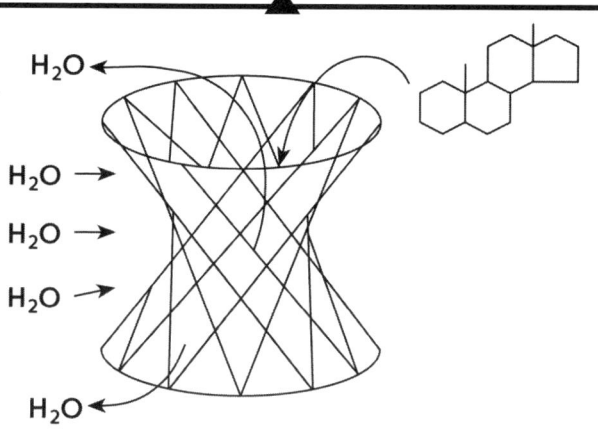

Fig. 3: Tunnel structure of matrix proteoglycans/glycosaminoglycans. Simultaneous transport of hydrophobic (lipophilic) substances in the interior of the tunnel and hydrophilic substances through binding to the exterior tunnel wall (guest-host complexing). The hyperbolic form is characteristic of minimal-energy surfaces. (17)

good lifestyle habits are very important in keeping the molecular sieve of the matrix clean. Glucose surpluses (due primarily to overconsumption of white flour and refined sugar) and age-related insulin resistance subject all components of the matrix, including the cellular glycocalyx, to nonenzymatic glycosylation, which is accompanied by the development of irreversible end products that cannot be broken down (the hormonal half-life of PG/GAGs is approximately 2 weeks).

Because peripheral vegetative nerve fibers terminate in the matrix, which also has access to the endocrine system via the capillaries, the matrix is directly linked to both the central nervous system and the centers in the brain stem and diencephalon that regulate the endocrine system (Figure 1). Thus, the matrix regulation system is also constantly influenced by psychological factors.

Fibroblasts (along with adipocytes and other related cells in bones, cartilage, and vascular walls) constitute the active center of matrix synthesis. In the central nervous system, neuroglial cells, which can synthesize matrix substances with the exception of collagen and elastin, perform both this function and immunosurveillance. On the body's periphery, the latter task is accomplished by cells of the unspecific immune system (macrophages, monocytes, dendritic cells, granulocytes), the regulatory immune system (Th3 lymphocytes), and the specific immune system (T and B lymphocytes).

The essential working principles of biological medicine are:

- Active involvement and deliberate exploitation of the body's self-regulating processes (autoregulation).
- Induction of self-healing (autonomic overcoming of diseases) through activation of autoregulatory processes (hygiogenetic principle).
- Indirect effects of therapeutically applied stimuli due to transmission of effects by the autoregulation system.
- Individual effects that depend on the nature of the stimulus and the patient's response status (stimulus-response principle).

These principles apply not only to naturopathy but also to homeopathy. They provide a model of scientific thinking that can explain many of the unique aspects of homeopathic medicine.

1.3.3 Inflammation as a Regulatory Principle

Only the extracellular matrix with its embedded cellular and neural components is capable of inflammation. Inflammation is a generalized response that does not point to any specific pathological process. Rather, such a process is characterized by interactions that are in part synergistic, in part antagonistic, and often redundant. Inflammation is significant in that it restores balance to disturbed regulatory relationships by eliminating "toxins" in the broadest sense (including, for example, psychological stress). Elimination is one aspect of detoxification. Ultimately, the goal is to reestablish autoregulation, i.e., the balance between catabolism and anabolism. A disturbance in this balance leads to an inflammatory reaction whose purpose is to readjust the autonomic nervous system. This means that any strain on the regulatory system (e.g., stress, environmental pollutants) causes the extracellular matrix to respond with increases in proinflammatory cytokines (e.g., tumor necrosis factor alpha [TNF-α]) and related molecules (chemokines such as macrophage-attracting proteins, adhesion molecules such as intercellular adhesion molecules [ICAMs]).

Concentrations of these proinflammatory molecules increase even in seemingly noninflammatory diseases such as mental illnesses or idiopathic vertigo. Patients experiencing myocardial infarction have been shown to have elevated ICAM-1 levels years before the acute episodes, while they were still clinically healthy. Such phenomena suggest that the ability of the extracellular matrix to develop inflammation is central to all regulatory processes.

All acquired chronic illnesses are preceded by long periods, even years, of health problems. Such problems constitute an appropriate field of activity for regulatory medicine. The outstanding effects of low- to mid-potency homeopathic remedies – and especially of antihomotoxic combination remedies – in cases of regulatory disturbance can be attributed not only to their detoxifying activity but also to the fact that they restore and maintain immunological tolerance via the so-called "immunological bystander reaction" (Figure 4).

In the immunological bystander reaction, specific single ingredients in the low- to mid-potency range (ca. 2X-14X, such as Bellis perennis 2X in Traumeel S or Toxicodendron quercifolium 4X in Zeel comp.) program a specific population of T lymphocytes to down-regulate proinflammatory lymphocytes (Th1 and Th2 lymphocytes) and upgrade humoral defense status by stimulating immunoglobulin-producing B lymphocytes. The theory of the bystander reaction is that when minute (potentized) and therefore nonimmunogenic quantities of soluble proteins in a homeopathic remedy are introduced into the body, they are endocytosed by macrophages and other antigen-presenting cells (APCs = monocytes and dendritic cells), which break them down internally into short chains of 5 to 15 amino acids ("motifs"). These motifs are transported back to the cell surface, where they are linked to major histocompatibility complexes (MHCs). Alternatively, this process may take place within a cell when new MHCs are synthesized, in which case the linked substances are transported to the cell surface together. T lymphocytes, attracted by a special chemokine produced by APCs, constantly patrol these cells, and the "fresh," immunogenically inexperienced or "naive" lymphocytes among them pick up the motifs and bind them to their own receptors. For this transfer of motifs to function, obviously the number of motifs presented to T-cell receptors must be as large and varied as possible. After binding the motifs,

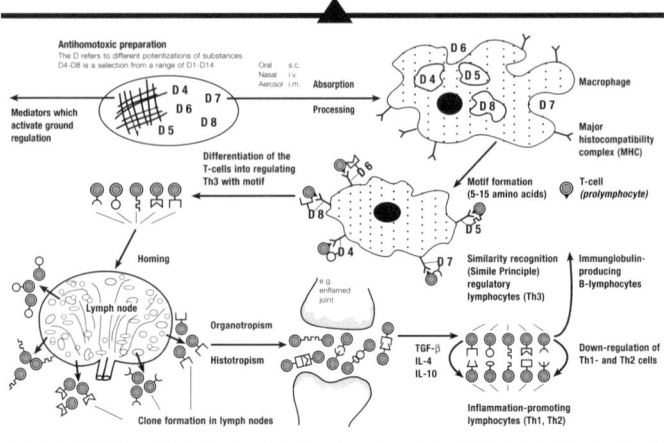

Fig. 4: The immunological bystander reaction. Low- to mid-potency single or combination homeopathic remedies induce development of regulatory lymphocytes (Th3 cells). After coming into contact with proinflammatory T lymphocytes (Th1 and Th2 cells), the Th3 cells release the anti-inflammatory cytokine TGF-β (transforming growth factor beta)

the lymphocytes metamorphose into regulatory Th3 lymphocytes, which are drawn to the site of inflammation by the organ-specific composition of chemotactic cytokines (chemokines). In the inflammation zone, inflammatory and regulatory lymphocytes compare the antigens with the motifs on their cell membranes. Establishing similarity is enough to stimulate the Th3 cells to produce anti-inflammatory cytokines (especially TGF-β), which down-regulate proinflammatory cytokines (TNF-α, interferon gamma [IFN-γ], interleukin 1 [IL-1]) until immunological tolerance is reestablished. TGF-β is also supported by IL-4 and IL-10 from Th-2 cells. Th2 cells also stimulate B cells to synthesize immunoglobulins.

Phytotherapeutic substances, which owe their immunomodulatory properties to their ability to stimulate an immunological bystander reaction, also play an important role in reestablishing immunological tolerance. Through proteolysis and hydrolysis in the small intestine, oral phytotherapeutic preparations are broken down to a stage comparable to low- to mid-potency homeopathic remedies, and the immunological bystander reaction is then triggered by macrophages in the epithelium of the small intestine. Endogenous molecules, which do not trigger an immune response, intensify the immunological bystander reaction when removed from the body and then reinjected (auto-sanguis therapy). The same is probably true of therapeutic use of the patient's own urine. It is important to remember that low concentrations or low- to mid-range potencies of substances communicate with cytokines and are therefore indispensable in maintaining immunological tolerance.

1.3.4 Latent Tissue Acidosis as an Obstacle to Therapy

Low- to mid-potency antihomotoxic combination medications, homeopathic remedies, phytotherapeutics, and alkalizing foods contain chemicals with unsaturated bonds (flavones, ubiquinone, pyrocatechins, etc.) that are capable of trapping excess free radicals. Until recently, the role that such medications and nutrients play in regulatory therapy by overcoming latent tissue acidosis has been underestimated.

Latent tissue acidosis is present in all persistent health problems (including chronic fatigue, low motivation, masked depression), as well as in chronic illnesses and tumors. It is the expression of increasing "rigidity" in matrix regulation and creates a proinflammatory situation.

Under normal circumstances, an antiport process occurs after every meal in the cells lining the gastric mucosa. Hydrochloric acid moves into the lumen of the stomach, while at the same time bicarbonate ions move in the other direction and are received by the underlying terminal capillaries. These ions are distributed to the extracellular matrix throughout the body, where they bind and mobilize excess acid valences, which are ultimately excreted in the urine. Consequently, the extracellular matrix becomes alkaline or neutral between meals, as reflected in the pH of the urine. This acid-base alternation can be supported or reestablished by administering bases or alkaline-forming foods as well as through elimination therapies (especially fasting) and the use of trace elements, vitamins, or orthomolecular medicine to capture free radicals. (It is important to remember that latent tissue acidosis is often accompanied by intestinal dysbiosis, which must be treated concurrently.) When "regulatory rigidity" occurs, 50% of metabolization takes place anaerobically, and the resulting development of lactic acid creates latent acidosis. The prospects of success for any therapy are poor if latent tissue acidosis is not recognized. If immunological tolerance can be reestablished, the health-promoting balance between the sympathetic and parasympathetic nervous systems can also be restored through autoregulation.

1.4 Reckeweg's Homotoxin Theory

Both Reckeweg's homotoxin theory and antihomotoxic therapy with homeopathic single and combination remedies are based on humoral pathology, that is, Reckeweg saw the organism as a fluid system (according to Bertalannfy) in the humoropathological sense. Substances flow in, react with and alter the organs of the fluid system and are altered by them, and ultimately leave the system. Tolerated substances produce no disturbance in the body's steady state, while toxic substances trigger defensive measures that are perceived as illness.

Beginning in 1948, Reckeweg developed the scientific concept of antihomotoxic therapy and homotoxicology. The first edition of his book *Homotoxins and Homotoxicoses* was published by Aurelia-Verlag, Baden-Baden (Germany), in 1952.

One of the fundamental concepts of homotoxin theory is that all manifestations of life, whether physiological or pathological, are subject to the laws of chemistry, i.e., predicated on conversions that can be understood in chemical terms.

Definition of Terms

Homotoxicology is an approach to medicine formulated by H.-H. Reckeweg. It is based primarily on homeopathy and also the matrix regulation system. The fundamental elements of homotoxicology are:
• The Arndt-Schulz law
• Von Bertalanffy's "steady state" principle
• S. Hahnemann's simile principle
• J. J. W. Lux's isopathic principle.

Homotoxicology combines elements of homeopathy, naturopathy, and conventional medicine.

Antihomotoxic medicine is a generic term encompassing the science of homotoxicology and the antihomotoxic therapy developed by H.-H. Reckeweg.

Antihomotoxic therapy is a holistic treatment concept based on the rules of homotoxicology. Its therapeutic objectives are:
▶ *Prevention* of illness
▶ *Detoxification* of organic systems
▶ *Regeneration* of organic systems
▶ *Symptom management*.

Prevention encompasses:
• Avoidance of toxins
• Therapeutic measures
• Maintaining health and a sense of well-being.

Detoxification encompasses
• Induction of excretion
• Elimination of homotoxins
• Activation of the organs of excretion such as the liver/gallbladder system, gastrointestinal tract, kidney/bladder system, lymphatic system, skin and mucous membranes, and the respiratory tract.

Regeneration encompasses
• Strengthening of organic functions
• Activation of cellular functions
• Immunomodulation.

Symptom management encompasses
• Positively influencing faulty regulation processes
• Causing symptoms to revert to the individual norm (regressive vicariation)
• Supporting the forces of spontaneous healing.

Homotoxins are all material (chemical/biochemical) and non-material (physical-energetic, psychological) influences that can cause health problems, i.e., the presence of these noxae causes regulatory disorders in the human body. Most diseases other than deficiency syndromes are due to the effects of homotoxins.

Homotoxins may be either exogenous or endogenous in origin. Table 4 presents one system of classifying homotoxins.

Modern medical science and environmental toxicology recognize that homotoxicoses can be triggered by many different noxae or contaminants. Table 5 lists typical examples of the factors enumerated in Table 4.

Endogenous and exogenous homotoxins
1. Physical factors
2. Chemical factors
   – inorganic
   – organic
3. Biological factors
4. Psychological factors

Tab. 4: Classification of homotoxins

Homotoxicosis is any pathophysiological condition caused by the effects of a homotoxin on cells and tissues. Homotoxicosis may appear on either the humoral or the cellular level and may induce morphological changes in tissues. Homotoxicosis triggers the organism's defense mechanisms, whose purpose is to either eliminate the homotoxins or to compensate for them and, when possible, to restore normal physiological conditions.

Health is the state in which both subjective perception and objective evidence confirm the absence of physical, mental, and emotional alterations and/or disorders.

Illness is any disorder of vital processes in individual organs or in the organism as a whole, accompanied by subjectively perceived and/or objectively detectable physical, mental, and/or emotional changes.

Healing. In conclusion, recovering from illness involves detoxifying and eliminating homotoxins and overcoming any damage they have caused.

Antihomotoxic therapy can be classified as natural because it uses only endogenous mechanisms. It attacks the true cause of ill-

Endogenous and exogenous homotoxins			
Physical factors	Chemical factors (inorganic/organic)	Biological factors	Psychological factors
• Weather and climate • Irradiation (light) • Noise • Radioactivity • Vibration • Color • Electromagnetic pollution and interference fields • Mechanical influences	• Contaminants in the air outside • Contaminants in the air inside buildings • Contaminants from air conditioners • VOC emissions (volatile organic compounds emitted by adhesives, floor coverings, insulation, packaging materials, coatings, paints, wallpaper, wood and other paneling, chipboard) • Cleaning products and sprays (surfactants) • Dust (carpets, paper, cigarette smoke) • Ozone • Gases • Chemicals • Medications	• Fungi • Bacteria • Viruses • Allergens • Endogenous intermediary products • Nutrition • Genetically manipulated foods	• Excessive stress • Lack of challenge • Social problems • Loss of love, insults, fear of loss • Lack of human communication • Harassment • Relationship problems, sexual problems • Pathological personality structures

Tab. 5: Typical examples of physical, chemical, biological, and psychological factors that can trigger homotoxicoses.

ness, namely, the toxins that provoke it. The biotherapeutic and antihomotoxic agents administered in antihomotoxic therapy (which may be either single or combination homeopathic remedies) stimulate and accelerate endogenous healing forces.

Organ system	HUMORAL PHASES		MATRIX PHASES		CELLULAR PHASES	
	Excretion Phases	Inflammation Phases	Deposition Phases	Impregnation Phases	Degeneration Phases	Dedifferentiation Phases
Skin	Episodes of sweating	Acne	Nevi	Allergy	Scleroderma	Melanoma
Nervous System	Difficulty concentrating	Meningitis	Cerebrosclerosis	Migraine	Alzheimer's disease	Gliosarcoma
Sensory System	Tears, otorrhea	Conjunctivitis, otitis media	Chalazion, cholesteatoma	Iridocyclitis, tinnitus	Macular degeneration, anosmia	Amaurosis, malignant tumor
Locomotor System	Joint pains	Epicondylitis	Exostosis	Chronic rheumatoid arthritis	Spondylosis	Sarcoma,
Respiratory Tract	Cough, expectoration	Bronchitis, acute	Silicosis, smoker's lung	Chronic (obstructive) bronchitis	Bronchiectasia, emphysema	Bronchial carcinoma
Cardiovascular System	Functional heart complaint	Endocarditis, pericarditis, myocarditis	Coronary heart disease	Heart failure	Myocardial infarction	Endothelioma
Gastrointestinal System	Heartburn	Gastroenteritis, gastritis	Hyperplastic gastritis	Chronic gastritis, malabsorption	Atrophic gastritis, cirrhosis	Stomach cancer, colon cancer
Urogenital System	Polyuria	Urinary tract infection	Bladder stones, kidney stones	Chronic urinary tract infection	Renal atrophy	Cancer
Blood	Reticulocytosis	Leucocytosis, suppuration	Polycythemia, thrombocytosis	Aggregation disturbance	Anemia, thrombocytopenia	Leukemia
Lymphatic System	Lymphedema	Lymphangitis, tonsillitis, lymphadenitis	Lymph-node swelling	Insufficiency of the lymphatic system	Fibrosis	Lymphoma, Hodgkin-/non-Hodgkin-Lymphoma
Metabolism	Electrolyte shift	Lipid metabolism disturbance	Gout, obesity	Metabolic syndrome	Diabetes mellitus	Slow reactions
Hormone System	Globus sensation	Thyroiditis	Goiter, adenoma	Hyperthyroidism, glucose intolerance	Menopausal symptoms	Thyroid cancer
Immune System	Susceptibility to infection	Weak immune system, acute infection	Weak reactions	Autoimmune disease, immunodeficiency, chronic infections	AIDS	Slow reactions
	Alteration*	Reaction*	Fixation*	Chronic Forms*	Deficits*	Decoupling*
Psyche	Functional psychological disturbance, 'nervousness'	Reactive depressive syndromes, hyperkinetic syndrome	Psychosomatic manifestation, neuroses, phobias, neurotic depression	Endogenous depression, psychosis, anxiety neurosis, organic psychosyndrome	Schizophrenic, defective states, mental deficiency	Mania, catatonia

BIOLOGICAL DIVISION

*Phase nomenclature in psychology.
The six-phase table is a field matrix reflecting medical experience based on careful observation and empirical learning.
It is a phase-by-phase arrangement of disorders with no direct relationship between them. No causal pathogenetic link between disorders can be inferred.
The structure of the table makes it suitable for developing a prediction system giving a better assessment of the possibilities for a vicariation effect.

Tab. 6: *Table of Homotoxicoses (Six-phase table) – Abridged version*

2. The Body's Defense against Homotoxins

2.1 The Body's Defense Possibilities

According to Reckeweg, illness is always a biologically meaningful process, the purpose of which is to eliminate endogenous or exogenous toxins and to repair, reduce, or contain the damage they cause. The type and degree of damage a homotoxin causes in the body depends on:

▶ the body's immune status, i.e., its regulatory capabilities, and
▶ the type of homotoxin and the duration and strength of its effect.

The body's initial attempts to eliminate the homotoxin are localized, limited, and acute. The very first defensive measure involves physiological elimination processes, which may be pathologically intensified to the point of inflammation. If this initial elimination effort fails, whether because of the structure of the homotoxin, the scope of its impact, the body's reduced reactivity (which may be due to iatrogenic damage, for example), or for any other reason, the body attempts to reduce the impact of the homotoxin by depositing it in specific tissues. Mesenchyme is the most frequent repository; other possibilities include fatty tissue, bile, and hair. Depending on the extent of the deposits and which tissue or organ is affected, a generalized disturbance of the body's regulatory capacity may result, often leading to chronic illness. If the disturbance is not rectified and the deposited toxins are not eliminated, cellular communication is disturbed and cell structures are damaged. This leads to structural changes in tissues and organs as the disease progresses, followed by degeneration and disintegration of affected tissue.

2.2 The Sequence of Responses

The body's defense against homotoxins proceeds in phases, which can be classified according to the following basic pathophysiological principles:

▶ Elimination
▶ Deposition
▶ Degeneration.

Each of these groups can be further differentiated into two subdivisions, as follows.

Elimination

1. In the **excretion phase**, the body's elimination functions are still able to remove the homotoxin. Options for elimination in this phase include both normal eliminations such as sweat, urine, feces, menses, and glandular secretions (bile) and intensified, semipathological forms of elimination such as hyperhidrosis, polyuria, and massive stools.
2. In the **inflammation phase**, physiological elimination of homotoxins is no longer possible. The greater defense system (see p. 40 ff.) is activated; pathological forms of elimination occur and may be associated with fever, inflammation, and pain (e.g., eczema, abscesses, boils).

Deposition

3. In the **deposition phase**, the homotoxin is removed from normally functioning cell associations and tissues and isolated in benign deposits such as lipomas, atheromas, dental calculus, and kidney, bladder, or gallstones. Clogging of the molecular sieve due to deposition of homotoxins in the extracellular matrix may create secondary symptoms, to which obesity and the like may also contribute. In the **impregnation phase**, pathological deposition of the homotoxin causes direct damage to cellular functions and structures, as in viral diseases, for example. This phase may remain latent and later give rise to a locus minoris resistentiae, or site of diminished resistance.

Degeneration

4. In the **degeneration phase**, intracellular structures are destroyed and breakdown products accumulate, disturbing organ function. Many chronic degenerative diseases such as cirrhosis, arthrosis, and sclerotic kidneys are manifestations of this phase.

5. In the **dedifferentiation phase**, structural changes in the genetic material in the cell nuclei and uncontrolled growth of affected tissue occur. This phase is characterized by malignant neoplasms and represents the body's last efforts to delay autointoxication for as long as possible.

From these successive phases, Reckeweg drew conclusions with regard to treatment and prognostication. He called the first three phases (excretion, inflammation, and deposition) *humoral phases.* In these phases, the principle of excretion predominates. Homotoxins are eliminated or isolated in the form of benign deposits. In most cases diseases with positive prognostication appear. Reckeweg contrasted the humoral phases with phases four through six (impregnation, degeneration, and dedifferentiation), which he called *cellular phases.* Here the principle of condensation predominates, and cell damage is triggered. Constitutional illnesses of dubious prognosis appear.

To clarify the fundamental qualitative distinction between humoral and cellular phases, Reckeweg introduced the concept of the *biological division*, a significant line of demarcation. To the left of the biological division, disturbances in the steady state are present but reversible and the body itself is able to compensate for them. Reversion to equilibrium can still be achieved, either through self-healing efforts or via targeted stimulation. Any disturbance to the right of the biological division has advanced to a point that makes compensation much more difficult or even, in some cases, completely impossible. Thus, only very limited reversibility of changes can be expected.

Table 7 summarizes the principles underlying each of these phases of illness.

| | Humoral Phases | | | Cellular Phases | | |
	• self-healing tendency • no damage to enzymes • excretion principle • favorable prognosis • environmental and constitutional factors			• deterioration of the patient's condition • damage to enzymes • condensation principle • dubious prognosis • constitutional factors		
Phase according to Reckeweg	Excretion phase	Inflammation phase	Deposition phase	Impregnation phase	Degeneration phase	Dedifferentiation phase
Chief principles	Alteration	Reaction	Fixation	Chronification	Deficits	Neoplasm formation
	Adequately functioning physiological elimination	Pathological elimination processes; activation of various defense functions (e.g., all inflammations)	Benign depositions of homotoxins; segregation of homotoxins from normally functioning cell associations and tissues	Damage to cellular functions and structures	Destruction of intracellular structures; accumulation of breakdown products	Structural changes in the genetic material in cell nuclei; uncontrolled growth of the affected tissue
Possible clinical manifestations	Health; early disturbances in homeostasis	Acute illnesses	Latent or subclinical illnesses; early stages of chronic illnesses	Chronic diseases; latent diseases	Chronic degenerative illness	Malignant neoplasm formation

Biological division

Tab. 7: Characteristics of the phases of homotoxicosis

In addition to classifying individual homotoxicoses (illnesses triggered by homotoxins) in terms of their different phases, Reckeweg derived a second dimension of his classification system from the effects of homotoxins on the different organ systems that develop out of different embryonic germ layers (Table 8). He considered the mesenchyme of fundamental importance, calling it and the three germ layers the most important tissues with regard to the body's response to homotoxins. Reckeweg found this two-dimensional classification system necessary because he had observed many cases in which the shift from one phase of illness to the next also involved a shift from one organ system to another, a shift that he attributed to movement of the homotoxin.

	Humoral Phases			Cellular Phases		
Organ system	Excretion phase	Inflammation phase	Deposition phase	Impregnation phase	Degeneration phase	Dedifferen- tiation phase
Skin						
Nervous system						
Sensory system						
Locomotor system						
Respiratory tract						
Cardiovascular system						
Gastrointesti- nal system						
Urogenital system						
Blood						
Lymphatic system						
Metabolism						
Hormone system						
Immune system						
Psyche						

Biological division

Tab. 8: Classification of homotoxicoses according to homotoxic phases and affected tissues.

2.3 The Six-Phase Table of Homotoxicoses

On the basis of these ideas, Reckeweg developed a differenti- ated graphic representation of the phases of homotoxicosis as they affect the different organ systems. Different stages of illness- es affecting various parts of the body can be classified according to this six-phase table (Table 9).

The Body's Defense against Homotoxins

Organ system	HUMORAL PHASES		MATRIX PHASES	CELLULAR PHASES		
	Excretion Phases	Inflammation Phases	Deposition Phases	Impregnation Phases	Degeneration Phases	Dedifferentiation Phases
Skin and Adnexae						
• Skin	Exanthema, episodes of sweating, desquamation	Acute mycosis, erysipelas; Acne, herpes simplex, diaper rash, varicella	Warts; Keratoderma, nevi, pruritus	Allergy; Contact eczema, psoriasis, seborrheic eczema, chronic mycosis, urticaria, neurodermatitis, pemphigus, lichen ruber	Decubitus ulcer, rosacea	Basalioma, melanoma, carcinoma
• Hair and nails		Folliculitis	Toxin storage	Onychomycosis	Alopecia	
• Subcutis	Sweat-gland disorder	Phlegmon, abscess	Atheroma, obesity	Cellulitis	Lupus erythematosus, scleroderma, vitiligo, cutaneous lymphoma	Lipoma
Peripheral and Central Nervous System	Neurasthenia, malaise, exhaustion, difficulty concentrating, lack of strength/energy	Headaches, dizziness, encephalitis, meningitis	Cerebrosclerosis	Convulsions, sleep disturbances, migraine, transient ischemic attack, dyslexia	Parkinson's disease, epilepsy, cerebral ischemia, disseminated encephalomyelitis, dementia, Alzheimer's disease	Neuroma, glioma, gliosarcoma, meningioma
• Peripheral nerves	Neurasthenia	Neuritis, lumbago, sciatica, neuralgia		Impulse conduction disturbance, chronic neuralgia, e.g., trigeminal neuralgia	Polyneuropathy, neurodystrophy	Neurofibromatosis
Sensory System						
• Eyes	Tears	Conjunctivitis, blepharitis, keratitis	Hordeolum, chalazion, vitreous opacity	Chronic conjunctivitis, uveitis, iridocyclitis	Sicca syndrome, cataract, retinitis pigmentosa, glaucoma, retinal detachment, macular degeneration	Blindness, malignant tumor
• Ears	Otorrhea, cerumen accumulation	Otitis media, otitis externa	Otosclerosis, cholesteatoma, otoliths	Tinnitus, labyrinthine vertigo	Impairment of hearing	Deafness, neoplasms

BIOLOGICAL DIVISION

Tab. 9: The six-phase table – long version

Tab. 9 Continued

Organ system	HUMORAL PHASES		MATRIX PHASES		CELLULAR PHASES	
	Excretion Phases	Inflammation Phases	Deposition Phases	Impregnation Phases	Degeneration Phases	Dedifferentiation Phases
• Sense of smell					Anosmia	
Locomotor System						
• Bone/cartilage	Bone disorder, cartilage disorder	Osteomyelitis	Exostosis, heel spur, osteoma	Soft-tissue rheumatism	Spondylosis; Osteoporosis, bone cysts, osteomalacia	Sarcomas; Chondroma
• Spinal column/joints	Joint pains, arthropathy, serous discharge	Rheumatoid arthritis, shoulder-arm syndrome, synovitis, periarthritis, epicondylitis	Periarthritis, calcarea	Chondropathy, chronic rheumatoid arthritis, cervicobrachial syndrome	Degenerative rheumatism, generalized osteoarthritis, disk prolapse, Bekhterev's disease	Osteosarcoma
• Connective tissue	Ligament disorder	Fibrositis, tendovaginitis	Gout, fibrosis, myogelosis	Fibromyalgia syndrome	Lower-leg ulcer	Fibroma, fibrosarcoma
• Muscles	Back disorder	Myalgia, myositis	Myogelosis	Soft-tissue rheumatism	Muscular atrophy	Myoma, myosarcoma
Respiratory Tract	Infection	Fever, influenza	Susceptibility to infections	Allergy		
• Throat, Nose, Ears	Epistaxis, rhinorrhea, cerumen accumulation, hypersalivation	Tonsillitis, sore throat, acute laryngitis, rhinopharyngitis, otitis media, otitis externa, sinusitis, tracheitis, herpes infection	Chronic rhinitis, candidiasis, tonsillar blockages, chronic sinusitis, tonsillar hypertrophy, abscess, adenoids	Allergic rhinitis, chronic rhinitis, aphthae, chronic tonsillitis, dizziness	Atrophic rhinitis, ozena, crypts	Leukoplakia, oral and lingual carcinoma lymphoma
• Bronchi	Cough, expectoration	Bronchitis, acute	Bronchopneumonia	Chronic (obstructive) bronchitis, asthma	Atelectasis, bronchiectasia, status asthmaticus	Bronchial carcinoma, mesothelioma
• Lungs	Dyspnea	Pneumonia	Silicosis, smoker's lung	Tuberculosis, alveolitis	Emphysema, pulmonary fibrosis	Lung cancer
Cardiovascular System	Circulatory disorder					
• Heart	Functional heart condition	Endocarditis, pericarditis, myocarditis	Coronary heart disease	Heart failure, hypertensive heart disease, extra-systoles, angina pectoris	Heart failure, cardiac arrhythmia, coronary heart disease, myocardial infarction, myocardiopathy	Endothelioma, rhabdomyosarcoma
• Arteries	Hypotensive dysregulation	Endarteritis	Peripheral vascular disease I, arteriosclerosis, embolism	Essential hypertension, hypotension, chronic, peripheral vascular disease II	Atrial fibrillation, atrial flutter, peripheral vascular disease III, arteriosclerosis	Endothelioma, peripheral vascular disease IV

BIOLOGICAL DIVISION (separating the Impregnation Phases from the Degeneration Phases)

Tab. 9 Continued

	HUMORAL PHASES		MATRIX PHASES		CELLULAR PHASES	
Organ system	Excretion Phases	Inflammation Phases	Deposition Phases	Impregnation Phases	Degeneration Phases	Dedifferentiation Phases
• Veins	Orthostatic syndrome	Phlebitis	Edema, thrombosis, thrombophlebitis	Venous valve insufficiency	Varices, hemorrhoids, crural ulcer	Endothelioma
• Lymph vessels	Lymph flow	Lymphadenitis	Edema, lymph-node swelling	Lymphatism	Elephantiasis	Lymphangiosarcoma, lymphoma
Gastrointestinal System						
• Teeth-mouth-jaws	Salivation	Glossitis, pulpitis, osteitis of the jaw, periodontitis	Granuloma	Allergy, Caries	Periodontosis	Leukoplakia, lingual and mucosal carcinoma
• Esophagus	Heartburn	Esophagitis	Achalasia	Cardiac insufficiency	Metaplasia	Esophageal cancer
• Stomach	Nausea, vomiting, dyspepsia	Gastroenteritis, gastritis	Hyperplastic gastritis	Chronic gastritis	Atrophic gastritis, gastric ulcer, peptic ulcer	Stomach cancer
• Duodenum		Gastroduodenitis			Duodenal ulcer	
• Small intestine	Diarrhea	Ileitis, jejunitis		Malabsorption, sprue	Malabsorption	
• Large intestine	Bloating, flatulence, diarrhea	Enteritis, colitis	Melanosis coli, constipation, candidiasis, polyposis coli	Irritable colon, ulcerative colitis, Crohn's disease	Diverticulosis	Colon cancer
• Liver-bile	Bile	Cholangitis, cholecystitis, hepatitis	Cholecystolithiasis, fatty liver	Liver function disturbance	Cirrhosis	Hepatocellular carcinoma, cholangioma
• Pancreas (excretory)		Pancreatitis	Siderosis	Chronic pancreatitis	Excretory pancreatic failure	Pancreatic cancer
Urogenital System						
• Kidneys	Polyuria	Pyelonephritis	Kidney stones	Nephrotic syndrome, chronic renal failure	Chronic renal failure renal atrophy	Kidney cancer, hyper-nephroma
• Bladder	Bladder disorder, irritable bladder	Cystitis, dysuria	Bladder stones	Dysuria, chronic urinary tract infection	Incontinence	Bladder cancer, bladder papilloma
• Sex organs	Leukorrhea, menstruation, mamillary secretion	Dysmenorrhea, prostatitis, orchitis, adnexitis, vaginitis myoma, ovarian cyst, and vulvo-vaginitis, candidiasis of the vulva/vagina	Prostatic hyp=rplasia,	Chronic prostatitis	Impotence, testicular atrophy, Peyronie's disease, atrophic vaginitis, sterility	Testicular cancer, prostate cancer, uterine cancer, ovarian cancer, cervical cancer
Blood				Disturbed fluidity balance, disturbed viscosity	Coagulation disturbance	

BIOLOGICAL DIVISION

Tab. 9 Continued

Organ system	HUMORAL PHASES		MATRIX PHASES		CELLULAR PHASES	
	Excretion Phases	Inflammation Phases	Deposition Phases	Impregnation Phases	Degeneration Phases	Dedifferentiation Phases
• Erythrocytes	Bleeding, reticulocytosis		Polycythemia		Anemia	
• Leukocytes	Leukocyte migration	Leukocytosis, suppuration	Abscess formation		Leukocytopenia	Leukemia
• Platelets			Thrombocytosis	Aggregation disturbance	Thrombocytopenia	
Lymphatic System	Lymphedema	Lymphangitis, tonsillitis, lymphadenitis	Lymph-node swelling	Insufficiency of the lymphatic system	Fibrosis	Lymphoma, Hodgkin-/non-Hodgkin lymphoma
Metabolism	Electrolyte shift	Lipid metabolism disturbance	Gout, obesity, hyperlipidemia	Metabolic syndrome	Iron-deficiency anemia, diabetes mellitus	Slow reactions
Hormone System	Endocrine disturbances				Menopausal symptoms	
• Hypothalamus/Pituitary gland			Pituitary adenoma			Acromegaly
• Thyroid	Globus sensation, hyperthyroidism	Thyroiditis	Goiter, adenoma	Hyperthyroidism, autoimmune thyroiditis	Hypothyroidism, nodular goiter	Thyroid cancer
• Pancreas (endocrine)		Acute pancreatitis		Glucose intolerance	Diabetes mellitus, pancreatic fibrosis	Insulinoma, glucagonoma
• Adrenals	Catecholamine secretion (stress)			Addison's disease, Cushing's disease	Adrenal atrophy	Adrenal cancer
Immune System	Susceptibility to infection	Weak immune system, acute infection	Weak reactions	Autoimmune disease, immunodeficiency, chronic infections	AIDS	Slow reactions
	Alteration*	Reaction*	Fixation*	Chronic forms*	Deficits*	Decoupling*
Psyche	Functional psychological disturbance, "nervousness"	Reactive depressive syndromes, hyperkinetic syndrome	Psychosomatic manifestation, neuroses, phobias, neurotic depression	Endogenous depression, psychosis, anxiety neurosis, organic psycho-syndrome	Schizophrenic defective states, mental deficiency	Mania, catatonia

BIOLOGICAL DIVISION

The Body's Defense against Homotoxins

2.4 The Vicariation Effect: Relationships and Shifts between Diseases

Because neural and humoral pathways connect all the cells of the body, the chemical transfer of homotoxins into one tissue necessarily affects other tissues. Thus, it makes sense that a shift from one phase of homotoxicosis to another may be accompanied by a shift to a different tissue (Figure 7). Reckeweg called this dual shift *vicariation* (from the Latin *vicarius* = substitute). Vicariation reflects changing symptoms due to displacement of illness-triggering toxins.

Although this recognition of vicariation is certainly not new, it gains new significance from the perspective of pinpointing phases of illness on the six-phase table. The direction and starting point of the shift in symptoms make it possible to judge whether the vicariation is biologically desirable. Students of homeopathy have long known that the course an illness takes demonstrates whether the patient's reaction is moving in the right direction, i.e., toward the possibility of complete recovery.

According to Hering's rule, the healing process moves:

▶ from vital organs and parts of the body to less important ones
▶ from the inside toward the outside
▶ from the top to the bottom
▶ in reverse chronological order (i.e., the symptoms that appeared last disappear first).

In contrast to this very general rule of homeopathy, Reckeweg's six-phase table allows detailed predictions with regard to the healing process. For example, in terms of Hering's rule, a shift in symptoms within the six-phase table may correspond to a shift from below to above or inside to outside. Locating the phases of an illness on Reckeweg's six-phase table, however, allows us to assess the course of the disease more specifically. The general rule is that shifts upward or to the left (regressive vicariation) indicate improvement, while shifts downward or to the right (progressive vicariation) indicate deterioration in the patient's condition.

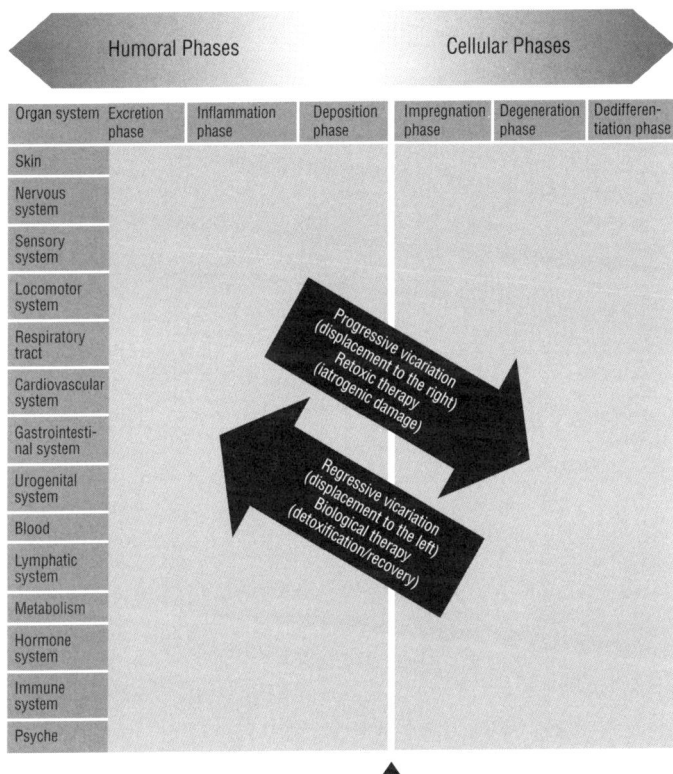

Organ system	Humoral Phases			Cellular Phases		
	Excretion phase	Inflammation phase	Deposition phase	Impregnation phase	Degeneration phase	Dedifferen- tiation phase
Skin						
Nervous system						
Sensory system						
Locomotor system						
Respiratory tract						
Cardiovascular system						
Gastrointesti- nal system						
Urogenital system						
Blood						
Lymphatic system						
Metabolism						
Hormone system						
Immune system						
Psyche						

Progressive vicariation (displacement to the right) Retoxic therapy (iatrogenic damage)

Regressive vicariation (displacement to the left) Biological therapy (detoxification/recovery)

Biological division

Fig. 7: Progressive and regressive vicariation

A frequently observed example of vicariation is the shift from eczema to asthma or vice versa. Depending on the patient's treatment and initial status, the change can occur in either direction (Figure 8).

The six-phase table also allows prognostication of complete recovery in different cases. The prognosis worsens steadily as moving through the phases from excretion to dedifferentiation. Harmless bodily reactions (such as perspiration) are located in the upper left corner while severe and generally incurable diseases (such as myosarcoma) are located in the lower right.

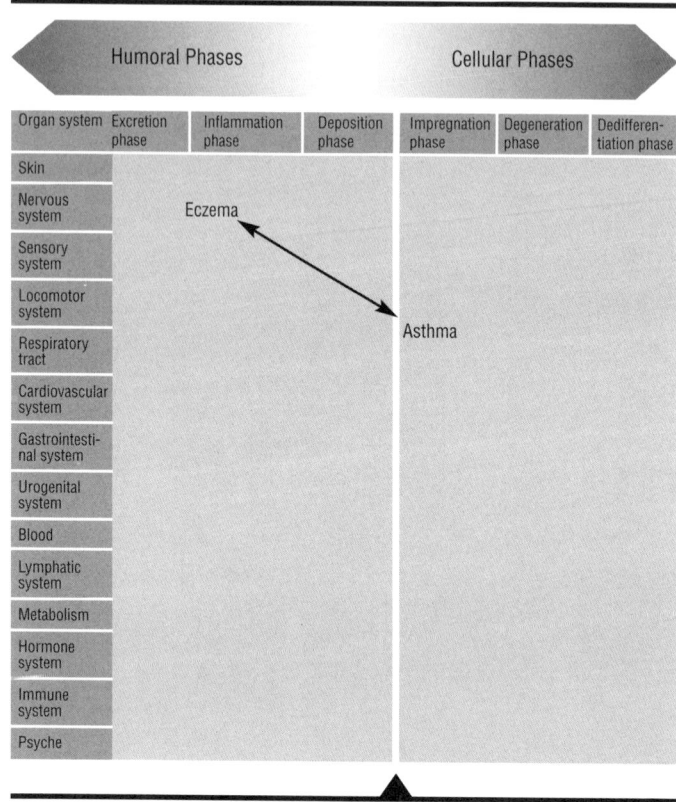

| Organ system | Humoral Phases | | | Cellular Phases | | |
	Excretion phase	Inflammation phase	Deposition phase	Impregnation phase	Degeneration phase	Dedifferen-tiation phase
Skin						
Nervous system		Eczema				
Sensory system						
Locomotor system						
Respiratory tract				Asthma		
Cardiovascular system						
Gastrointesti-nal system						
Urogenital system						
Blood						
Lymphatic system						
Metabolism						
Hormone system						
Immune system						
Psyche						

Biological division

Fig. 8: An example of vicariation

2.5 Accumulation and Displacement of Homotoxins

Reckeweg described a phenomenon in which homotoxins that are ready to be eliminated instead accumulate and shift completely to a different tissue as a consequence of some therapeutic measure, for example. In this instance, the homotoxins generally do not undergo further chemical change.

2.6 The Retoxic Effect

All cellular phases are characterized by damage to substances within the cells, but not all such phases are consequences of homotoxin activity, regardless of how prolonged or massive. Cellular phases are often induced when biologically meaningful endogenous processes such as fever or inflammation, which are essentially attempts to detoxify and eliminate homotoxins, are interrupted or totally suppressed. Reckeweg called this phenomenon the *retoxic effect*. In such cases, structural damage to cells initially produces a locus minoris resistentiae, or site of diminished resistance, which persists in a latent stage. This phenomenon is evident in some impregnation-phase diseases.

2.7 Evasive Phases

In certain cases, biologically more desirable phases exist concurrently with either manifest or latent cellular phases (Figure 9). For example, an inflammation phase may continually eliminate endogenous homotoxins and thus hold a degenerative-phase disease at bay, to a certain extent. An evasive phase serves as a biological safety valve of sorts and should be allowed to run its course unhindered, since suppressing it would destroy the patient's relatively labile equilibrium, allowing the illness to manifest fully or to worsen. Excretion, inflammation, and deposition phases can all function as evasive phases.

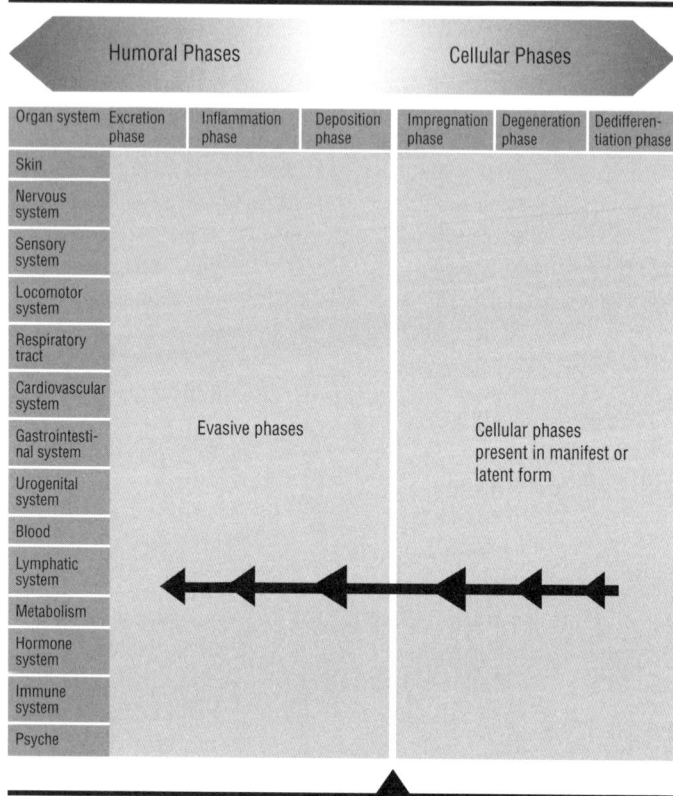

Fig. 9: Evasive phases

2.8 The Greater Defense System

In the human or animal body, a sophisticated system of inter-connected defensive mechanisms is available to eliminate toxins and repair damage. With the help of these mechanisms, homotoxins are either eliminated or combined with other substances to form harmless compounds called *homotoxons*. In homotoxicology, this entire system of detoxification mechanisms is called the *greater defense system*. It consists of five subsystems (Figure 10).

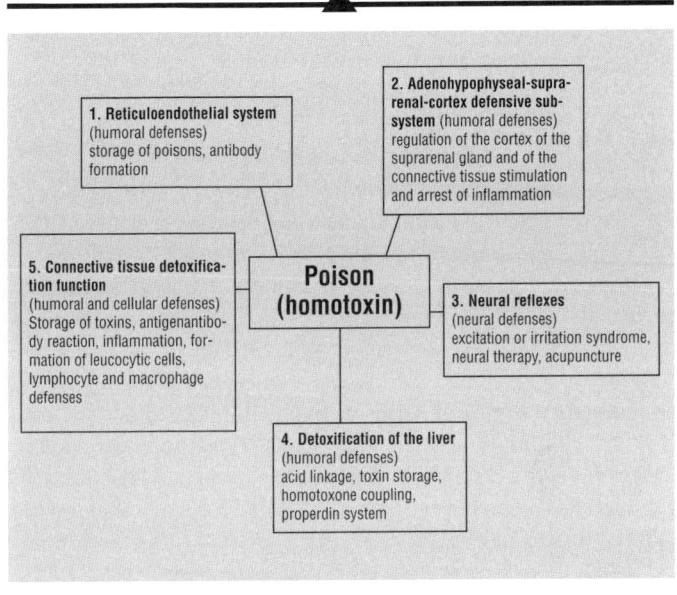

Fig.10: The greater defense system.

2.8.1 The Reticuloendothelial System (RES)

The reticuloendothelial system, also known as the lymphoreticular system, is an essential part of the body's unspecific defenses. It consists of a heterogeneous group of cells that originate in the bone marrow and are distributed throughout the body. They appear first in the blood as monocytes. In the form of macrophages, they then move into various tissues and organs, where they are given different names (e.g., Kupffer cells in the liver, alveolar macrophages in the lungs, histiocytes in connective tissue). The tasks of the RES are to eliminate foreign particles, to assist in antibody formation, and to synthesize and release biologically active substances (complement factors, lysosomal enzymes, prostaglandins, TNF, IFN-γ, etc.).

Through its role in inducing synthesis of specific antibodies, the RES is also closely linked to specific immunity. Mayr says of the interactions between specific and unspecific immunity, "The immune system, rather than being linear, is highly interconnected and subject to a biological steady state. Paraspecific and specific immune activities, therefore, are interdependent, control each other, and can metamorphose from one into the other." (21)

2.8.2 The Adenohypophysis-Adrenal Cortex Mechanism

Regulation of inflammatory processes is possible because of the adenohypophysis-adrenal cortex mechanism. During inflammation, the hormones of this axis intervene more strongly in the physiological circadian alternation of acids and bases in the connective tissue. The adenohypophysis is activated by dissolved (humoral), vegetative (autonomic), or peripheral (homotoxins) stimuli. Hoff explained the induction of this central response to inflammatory stimuli in terms of mobilizing the autonomic nervous system, but today this induction can also be understood in terms of Selye's universal adaptation syndrome. The release of growth hormone enhances connective tissue function with regard to inflammation and tissue renewal.

In addition to growth hormone, the adenohypophysis also releases adrenocorticotropic hormone, which stimulates the adrenal cortex to release glucocorticoids that suppress inflammatory reactions by inhibiting mesenchymal processes such as fibroblast growth and vascularization in inflammatory tissue.

2.8.3 Neurological Defense against Toxins

When a substance with homotoxic effects contacts nerve endings, reflex-like responses are triggered. These responses influence regulation variables such as blood pressure, vessel diameter, and muscle tone. Tissue and cell functions are intensified (as they are in inflammation) to enhance homotoxin elimination. Reckeweg calls this phenomenon *excitation syndrome*. When a stimulus is too strong or too prolonged, an *irritation syndrome* develops, in which reflex cascades may cause damage even in remote parts of the body.

2.8.4 Liver Detoxification

The central importance of the liver as an organ of detoxification in intermediary metabolism is well known. In the liver, metabolites and exogenous substances introduced by foods or medications are chemically changed through oxidation, hydroxylation, or conjugation with other substances such as glucuronides or sulfates. Every liver cell is capable of breaking down or transforming more than a thousand different substances. Coupling homotoxins with other substances produces either compounds that can then be eliminated or substances that no longer have toxic effects (homotoxons).

2.8.5 The Protective Function of Connective Tissue

Connective tissue constitutes an extensive drainage system that receives both nutrients and metabolic wastes and either stores them temporarily or moves them out through the lymph and blood vessels. The circadian acid-base rhythm causes natural alternation in connective tissue between storage phases (when the milieu is alkaline) and evacuation phases (when the milieu is acidic). Connective tissue may also store waste products that cannot be converted or eliminated immediately. These substances must be broken down later by means of an inflammation phase.

As a temporary or final repository for many different exogenous and endogenous chemicals, connective tissue is an important component of the greater defense system. Its purpose within that system is to remove harmful substances from the body's metabolic circulation to maintain homeostasis.

Many details of the detoxification processes that occur in cases of specific homotoxin loading remain unexplained. The greater defense system, however, with its five interconnected and interacting subsystems, offers a sound basis for further observation and research in this field. The concept of the greater defense system, which emphasizes the links between the immune system and other systems in the body, provides homotoxicology with a very comprehensive understanding of the body's self-protective mechanisms. This concept is in harmony with the results of the most recent research. Says Mayr, "Conventional ideas about the autonomy of the immune system and its responses are no longer tenable. The immune system is not only highly configured internally and linked to a network of interdependent regulatory mechanisms that stimulate or repress it, but it also reacts with other essential dynamic systems in the body such as the endocrine, metabolic, and nervous systems. The result is a fateful feedback control system that is subject to a biological steady state. Only in recent years has our understanding of this phenomenon begun to grow as a result of comparative research, interdisciplinary cooperation, and a great deal of empirical observation." (21)

3. The Status of Homotoxicology

This chapter will describe homotoxicology's relationship to homeopathy, links to conventional medicine, and significance within the broader field of holistic medicine.

From 1948 onward, Dr. Hans-Heinrich Reckeweg pioneered homotoxicology as a scientific school of thought and antihomotoxic therapy as its practical application. During his long years of practice as a homeopathic physician, he observed that the medications of the classic homeopathic materia medica have little effect on some chronic illnesses, especially those involving severe organ and tissue defects. He also recognized an additional problem, namely, the increasing variety of damages due to general environmental toxicity. Reckeweg incorporated therapeutic and scientific observations and insights from the fields of biochemistry, pathology, physiology, and toxicology into the science of homotoxicology, which he described as an expanded version of homeopathy or homeotherapy.

The initial cause of illness, the body's response to this cause, the different forms of illness that a single cause may trigger, and the transformation of one illness into another are all explained by Reckeweg's homotoxin theory, which resulted in both a more profound and comprehensive understanding of the concept of illness and, on the practical level, the development of antihomotoxic therapeutic agents. These agents' quasi-antigenic stimulating effects mobilize latent defense mechanisms against newly introduced toxins. Since Reckeweg's time, a great deal of clinical and experimental evidence, compiled in part in university clinics, has documented and verified the efficacy of antihomotoxic biotherapeutic preparations.

Table 10 presents the differences among classic homeopathy, homotoxicology, and allopathic medicine in terms of modern pharmacotherapy.

In a dissertation entitled *The Concept of Chronic Illness in H.-H. Reckeweg's Homotoxin Theory: Differences and Commonalities in Comparison to the Ideas of Conventional and Biological Medicine*, Abel defines the term "chronic illness" from the per-

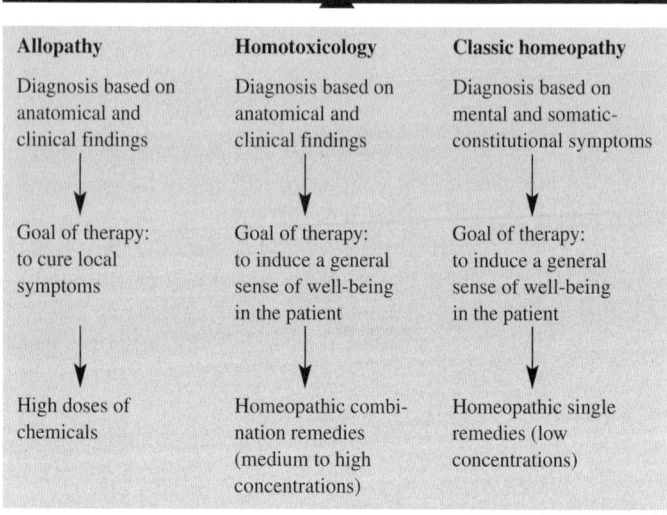

Allopathy	Homotoxicology	Classic homeopathy
Diagnosis based on anatomical and clinical findings	Diagnosis based on anatomical and clinical findings	Diagnosis based on mental and somatic-constitutional symptoms
↓	↓	↓
Goal of therapy: to cure local symptoms	Goal of therapy: to induce a general sense of well-being in the patient	Goal of therapy: to induce a general sense of well-being in the patient
↓	↓	↓
High doses of chemicals	Homeopathic combi-nation remedies (medium to high concentrations)	Homeopathic single remedies (low concentrations)

Tab. 10: Distinctions among different schools of therapy (Bianchi)

spective of homotoxicology as well as from conventional and holistic viewpoints (as represented by the pathologists Sandritter and Pischinger, respectively). Sandritter's static view of illness equates both illness and clinical findings with visible morphological change. In this view, illness is a condition rather than a process, and the goal of therapy is to eliminate symptoms, although defects frequently persist after healing. Reckeweg's therapy aims at comprehensive regeneration. For Reckeweg, illness is a dynamic, responsive process in which the changes visible at any moment may quickly alter, intensify, or disappear. Very different illnesses may in fact be related through what Reckeweg called the vicariation effect; that is, one illness is transformed into another when the homotoxin shifts into a different tissue.

According to Abel, Reckeweg's homotoxin theory and Pischinger's matrix regulation system have much in common. In contrast to Sandritter, these authors share a holistic view of illness in which the basic mesenchyme functions (maintaining equilibrium and defending the body against noxae) play a central role. The difference between Reckeweg's and Pischinger's theories lies primarily in Reckeweg's inclusion of aspects of cellular pathology, allowing distinctions among humoral and cellular diseases involving different pathophysiological processes, while Pischinger's model always equates illness with a matrix regulation disturbance and therefore does not recognize subdivisions into different types of illness. According to Abel, the fact that both authors see therapy as directed not toward specific organs but toward a generalized (i.e., holistic) regeneration of the organism illustrates the close relationship between their theories.

Furthermore, Abel describes the varied and extensive ways in which Reckeweg's homotoxin theory is linked to both Sandritter's cellular pathology model and Pischinger's theory of humoral pathology. Abel demonstrates in detail that Reckeweg occupies a middle ground between these other two, although admittedly homotoxicology stands closer overall to holistic medicine (and thus to Pischinger) than to Sandritter's conventional medicine.

Another important point is that in conventional medicine, the distinction between acute and chronic illness has no specific consequences for therapy, and Pischinger's system also does not distinguish between them. In contrast, Reckeweg's homotoxin theory incorporates several conclusions that strictly delineate acute symptoms from chronic disease processes. First, an acute illness may serve a positive, useful purpose, either as a means of preventing full manifestation of a chronic condition or as the expression of a therapeutically desirable retrogression (Reckeweg's *regressive vicariation*) from a chronic to a less serious form of illness. Second, acute symptoms may represent an evasive phase that attempts to circumvent an underlying chronic illness although it cannot eliminate it. In such cases, metabolic "emergency exits" serve as safety valves that prevent more serious manifestations of disease, such as malignant degeneration.

It is not surprising that conventional medical therapy continues to experience increasing therapeutic failures, especially in cases of chronic, allergic, or immunological illnesses, or that it sometimes causes irreparable secondary organic damage. Diagnostics as practiced today proceeds according to strict criteria that depend on the use of technology and laboratory testing, with the goal of verifying pathological and etiological factors in one or more diseased organ systems. The patient is not seen as a totality encompassing psychological, social, phenotypic, and constitutional characteristics in addition to organic damage. Although the use of high doses of allopathic medications administered on a symptomatic basis generally results in subjective freedom from symptoms, in actuality symptom suppression often leads either to chronic illness (Reckeweg's *progressive vicariation*) or to iatrogenic secondary illness, significantly reducing the patient's chances for a complete and lasting recovery. Table 11 presents the essential differences between conventional medicine and homeopathy.

	Conventional medicine	Homeopathy
Theory of disease	Etiological	Phenomenological
Therapeutic research	Deductive	Inductive
Therapy	Antagonistic and substitutive	Regulatory
Therapeutic method	Biochemical change	Feedback adjustment
Dosage	High	Low
Adverse effects	Frequent	Seldom
Drug-induced damage	Frequent	Never
Guiding principle	Generalization	Individualization

Tab. 11: Differences between conventional medicine and homeopathy. (12)

Conventional medicine, with the help of scientific knowledge, attempts to standardize and objectify disease processes by applying uniform conventions. In contrast, biological medicine's holistic perspective personalizes the problem of illness, explores the interrelationships among symptoms and their relationship to the environment, and replaces conventional medicine's normative understanding of disease with individualized perspectives of each patient's illness. In antihomotoxic therapy, also a holistic theory, the three domains of disease classification, diagnosis, and therapy form the basis of a profound understanding of health and illness.

Most diseases today involve functional disorders and/or failure of regulatory systems. Chronic illnesses in particular are expressions or consequences of long-term disturbances in autoregulatory processes.

Conventional medicine does not sufficiently acknowledge the importance of regulatory processes for therapy. If spontaneous healing can be understood as the result of regulatory processes, however, it would seem obvious to utilize natural regulatory measures when therapeutic intervention is needed to produce a cure. Holistic therapeutic measures aim to restore the function of disturbed feedback control loops.

When a feedback loop is disturbed and spontaneous healing does not occur, three types of therapeutic intervention are possible:

▶ attempting to eliminate the cause of illness or prevent its effects (causal therapy = eliminating the disturbance variable)
▶ attempting to relieve or suppress the symptoms of illness (passive symptomatic therapy = altering the regulative pathway)
▶ influencing the body's self-regulation to support or stimulate self-healing tendencies (reactivation therapy = eliminating the disturbance and/or control parameter).

All reactivation therapies function according to the principle that the smallest effective (and preferably subliminal) stimulus is best. Reactivation therapies that bring order into disturbed regulatory systems and stimulate endogenous regulation in the direction of self-healing can be considered holistic therapeutic measures.

The "biocybernetic model" (Figure 11) graphically illustrates the principles of the holistic viewpoint. This model begins with regulatory systems in which the smallest functional entity is the

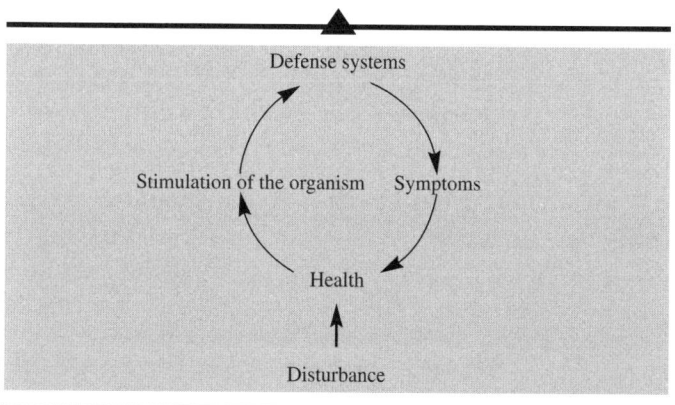

Fig. 11: The biocybernetic model. (14)

feedback control loop. At this level, we distinguish a regulation variable, a regulatory mechanism, and afferent and efferent branches of the loop. In this instance, health is the regulation variable and defense regulation systems constitute the regulatory mechanism.

In this model, illness and recovery are understood as follows. A disturbance variable affects a regulation variable, causing deviation of the actual value from the desired value. This process works via the afferent branch of the regulatory system to supply information to the regulatory mechanism, which responds via the efferent branch with attempts to make the actual value equal the desired value.

Homotoxicology attempts to either strengthen or adjust the organism's autoregulation.

Reckeweg intended homotoxicology to unite conventional medicine with the perspectives of holistic forms of therapy (especially homeopathy). He integrated the essential and fundamental demands of both disciplines into his theoretical model and reaped great practical benefits as a result.

4. Antihomotoxic Biotherapeutic Medications

4.1 Homotoxicology's Consequences for Pharmacotherapy

With regard to therapy, the most important conclusion that can be drawn from homotoxicology's teleological approach to disease is that therapeutic efforts must not hinder but instead must aim to activate and support endogenous defense mechanisms. As a rule, conventional pharmaceuticals fail to meet these requirements and in fact often cause additional stress on the organism by blocking the natural course of specific and non-specific immune responses. Furthermore, metabolizing allopathic medications, which are generally administered at much higher doses, require great expenditures of energy. For example, 1 g of acetylsalicylic acid (molecular weight, 180.2) contains approximately 5.5 nmol or 10 (20) molecules. This means that each of the approximately 10 (14) cells of the human body is impacted by a million molecules of the active ingredient if it is equally distributed, and even more if concentrations vary.

To support the body's defensive efforts without compounding the problems caused by toxins already present, homotoxicology works with the weak stimuli that are characteristic of homeopathic therapy. Because function-stimulating and regulatory medications such as homeopathic and biotherapeutic antihomotoxic agents deliberately exploit endogenous mechanisms, the effects of such medications are qualitative and, as a rule, not dose-dependent in the modern pharmacotherapeutic sense. The success of therapy is generally much more dependent on the patient's compliance with an individually prescribed treatment plan (see Chapter 5) than on dosage. As a rule, therefore, identical dosages may be prescribed for most patients.

The medications of the homeopathic materia medica, with their regulatory effects and weak stimuli, are the mainstays of antihomotoxic therapy. However, successful treatment of a great variety of illnesses requires an expansion of the classic homeopathic repertory (which includes substances of mineral, plant, and animal origin, plus nosodes). Modern biochemical research provides the foundation for homotoxicological use of additional classes of medications (intermediary catalysts, homeopathically adjusted allopathic remedies, and suis-organ preparations), which are often administered according to the Aequalia principle of isotherapy or isopathy (*aequalia aequalibus*), meaning that therapy uses the same substances that trigger the illness.

A large part of the antihomotoxic repertory consists of medications in which substances either of different potencies or from different classes are combined. In homotoxicology, illness is understood as the consequence of multiple factors that can be targeted by combination medications whose ingredients intervene on different levels. Thus, combining the effects of different substances that work toward the same end (such as single-constituent preparations with similar cardinal symptoms, different potencies of a single-constituent preparation, nosodes, or suis-organ preparations) is an important therapeutic principle in homotoxicology.

On another level, the fact that the specific and non-specific immune systems are inextricably linked and work together to eliminate homotoxins also confirms the principle of combining working mechanisms. Likewise, to elicit healing in the homotoxicological sense, the action of all prescribed medications should complement the body's attempts at self-healing. For these reasons, deliberately combining remedies that work in the same direction is both natural and advantageous.

4.2 Definition of Terms and Classification of Antihomotoxic Preparations

The medications administered in antihomotoxic therapy contain very diverse ingredients. One proven method of classification recognizes the following classes of antihomotoxic medications.

▶ **Combination Preparations**, which include these sub-groups:
Specialties
Homaccords
Mixed Injeels
Composita Preparations

All of these medications combine ingredients drawn from the entire palette of substances used in antihomotoxic medications. The remedies known as *specialties* are distinguished by their one-word trade names such as "Zeel" or "Engystol", while the other groups have names ending in "Homaccord", "Injeel", or "Compositum."

The specialties and the mixed injeels were the first antihomotoxic medications developed. The specialties have always been available in a variety of forms, while mixed injeels are available only in ampules that can be used for injection. In contrast, the homaccord preparations were originally available only as orally administered drops, but ampules have been added for parenteral administration.

The composita preparations, introduced into the antihomotoxic repertory during 1973 to 1976, represent a later development in antihomotoxic medications.

▶ **Single-Constituent Homeopathic Preparations**
This class can be further subdivided into "single-constituent preparations in potency chords" (injeels) and "single-constituent preparations in single potencies" (special preparations). All medications in these two groups are named after the homeopathic remedy they contain. "Injeel" or "Injeel forte" is appended to the remedy name of a potency chord, while the potency level is added to the name of each single-potency remedy. However, the single-constituent preparations in potency chords, or injeels, are legally classified as combination medications.

▶ **Homeopathically Adjusted Allopathic Remedies**
The medications in this class contain conventional allopathic medications that have undergone further processing according to the guidelines of the German homeopathic pharmacopoeia (HAB) to make them available in homeopathic (potentized) form.

▶ **Intermediary Catalysts**
These medications contain substances that play important roles as metabolites or catalysts in intermediary metabolism, especially in the citric acid cycle and cellular respiration.

▶ **Nosodes**
Nosodes are homeopathic preparations of pathologically altered tissues, disease by-products, or microorganisms. They do not contain live pathogens or other materials that could transmit disease.

▶ **Suis-Organ Preparations**
The raw materials for these medications are obtained from healthy pigs. The effects of the suis-organ preparations are regenerative and vitalizing on the cellular level.

These four classes of medications, whose production and use are described in detail below, are administered primarily in the form of potency chords. Because a mixture of different potencies of a single ingredient is considered a combination medication under German law, almost all antihomotoxic medications, not only those specifically designated as combination remedies, are officially combination medications. Only the group of single-constituent preparations in single potencies, which can be produced from almost any of the ingredients of antihomotoxic medications, can be called single-constituent preparations both legally and in the common parlance of homeopathy.

Despite these complications, the classifications used above will be retained for purposes of the more detailed discussion of antihomotoxic medications that follows.

Table 11 gives an overview of these four classes of medications, which are more or less specific to homotoxicology.

Class of Medications	Mode of Action	Preferred Applications
Homeopathically Adjusted Allopathic Remedies	Stimulation of endogenous forces of healing to overcome drug-induced damage	Treatment of damage due to allopathic medications
Intermediary Catalysts	Stimulation of disturbed cellular and enzymatic functions by administering homeopathic concentrations of physiological metabolic substrates, vitamins, and coenzymes	Chronic illnesses involving blockage of cellular functions such as enzyme functions in the respiratory chain
Nosodes	Stimulation of defense mechanisms to eliminate toxin-induced damages due to past infections	Chronic disease states related to past infections
Suis-Organ Preparations	Stimulation of disturbed organ functions by means of homeopathic (potentized) organ extracts	Chronic and degenerative diseases involving specific organs

Tab.11: An overview of substances used in antihomotoxic therapy (other than substances included in the classic homeopathic materia medica)

4.3 Classes of Antihomotoxic Medications

This section describes the individual classes of preparations used in antihomotoxic therapy.

4.3.1 Combination Preparations

Because homotoxicology attributes great significance to the principle of synergy, this class includes the most widely used preparations in the antihomotoxic repertory.

In as much as they contain ingredients common to homeopathy, the development of combination formulas that target specific clinical diseases or syndromes is based either on cardinal symptoms known from the drug pictures of individual ingredients or on well-established indications. Reckeweg, who developed most of these medications, was an expert on the homeopathic materia medica. He was aware of the relationships among remedies and experienced in administering single-constituent preparations in combination. Antihomotoxic combination medications can be prescribed successfully according to clinical indications. Familiarity with the theory behind homeopathic remedies is very helpful, however, because practitioners who are familiar with the drug pictures and unique symptoms of the ingredients are better able to individualize the use of the combination (see Chapter 5).

Antihomotoxic combination remedies can be divided into the following four subgroups: specialties, homaccords, mixed injeels, and composita preparations.

Specialties

Specialized antihomotoxic medications such as Gripp-Heel (Table 10), Traumeel, Zeel, and Vertigoheel are fixed combinations of homeopathic single-constituent preparations (generally in only one potency each). These preparations target specific clinical diseases or syndromes and are administered according to homeopathic cardinal symptoms or well-established indications. These medications may be available in one or more forms (injectable solution, ointments, suppositories, tablets, or drops).

▲

Gripp-Heel (tablets)
Composition:
3 plant-derived ingredients, as single potencies
  Aconitum napellus 4X (garden monkshood)
  Bryonia cretica 4X (red bryony)
  Eupatorium perfoliatum 3X (common boneset)
1 animal ingredient, as a single potency
  Lachesis 12X (bushmaster snake venom)
1 mineral ingredient, as a single potency
  Phosphorus 5X (white phosphorus)

Tab.12: Example of the composition of a specialty preparation

Homaccords

Homaccord solutions combine two or more homeopathic ingredients, each in both high and low potencies (potency chords). Typically, the potency levels are 2X–6X, 10X, 30X, 200X, and sometimes 1000X (see Table 11). Potency chords were first mentioned in 1913 by the Spanish physician Cahis.(4) Their therapeutic impact is consistently both broader in scope and more profound than that of single potencies. Julian also reported on the use of mixtures of different potencies of the same homeopathic remedy, in his case a nosode.18 Taking the earlier work of Cahis, Castueil, Barishac, Fortier-Bernoville, and others as his basis, Julian described the effects of such a mixture as "faster, deeper, longer-lasting, and associated with fewer side effects". (18) Experience has demonstrated that single potencies retain their unique effects even when mixed in potency chords, so that the resulting effect is not merely the average of the different potencies. Experience in veterinary medicine in particular confirms that potency chords address not only organic and functional disturbances but also behavioral disorders, which are otherwise thought to be influenced only by high potencies. The high potencies of homaccords also make them very useful in treating chronic illnesses.

The fact that the solution contains low, middle, and high potencies reduces the possibility of overreaction. Initial aggravation or side effects are almost never observed when homaccords are administered.

Any homaccord can be used either alternately or together with any other homaccord or other oral or injectable Heel bio-therapeutic medication.

Homaccords were first made available in the form of drops for oral administration but were later also marketed as ampules for parenteral administration. In the ampule homaccords, the base potencies of the individual ingredients are generally two to three levels higher than they are in the liquid preparations.

▲

Apis-Homaccord (drops)
Composition:
2 animal ingredients in the form of potency chords
 Apis mellifica 2X, 10X, 30X, 200X, 1000X (honeybee)
 Apisinum 6X, 30X (bee venom)
1 plant ingredient in the form of a potency chord
 Scilla 2X, 10X, 30X (sea onion, spring squill)
1 mineral ingredient in the form of a potency chord
 Tartarus stibiatus 2X, 10X, 30X, 200X (tartar emetic)

Tab.13: Example of the composition of a homaccord

Mixed Injeels

Like the homaccords, the medications known as injeels (Angio-Injeel, Circulo-Injeel, Injeel-Chol, Metro-Adnex-Injeel, Neuralgo-Rheum-Injeel, Neuro-Injeel ampules, Tonico-Injeel, to list a few examples) also contain several ingredients in the form of potency chords (see Table 12). Despite this similarity in composition, however, the mixed injeels are considered a separate group because they were originally offered in forms suitable for parenteral administration. The distinction between the two groups of preparations persists, especially since the different endings on their names makes them easy to distinguish. The effects and preferred uses of mixed injeels are the same as those of homaccords. Unlike the latter, however, the mixed injeels are still available only in injectable form (ampules).

Metro-Adnex-Injeel (ampules)
Composition:
3 animal ingredients in the form of potency chords
Apis mellifica 10X, 30X, 200X (honeybee)
Lachesis 10X, 30X, 200X, 1000X (bushmaster snake venom)
Crabro vespa 10X, 30X, 200X (hornet)
4 plant ingredients in the form of potency chords
Lilium tigrinum 10X, 30X, 200X (tiger lily)
Lycopodium 10X, 30X, 200X, 1000X (club moss)
Pulsatilla 10X, 30X, 200X, 1000X (windflower)
Cimicifuga 10X, 30X, 200X (bugbane)
1 mineral ingredient in the form of a potency chord
Hydrargyrum bichloratum 10X, 30X, 200X (mercuric chloride)

Tab.14: Example of the composition of a mixed injeel

Composita Preparations

Some composita preparations, such as Cantharis compositum S (Table 15) and Carbo compositum, consist exclusively of single potencies of ingredients drawn from the materia medica of classic homeopathy.

Cantharis compositum S (ampules)
Composition:
1 animal ingredient in the form of a single potency
Cantharis (Lytta vesicatoria) 4X (Spanish fly)
3 mineral ingredients in the form of single potencies
Arsenicum album 8X (white arsenic)
Mercurius solubilis Hahnemanni 8X
Hepar sulfuris 8X

Tab. 15: Example of the composition of a composita preparation consisting of ingredients drawn from classic homeopathy

More often, however, composita preparations also include ingredients from the classes of medications that are more or less specific to homotoxicology, as is the case, for example, with Solidago compositum S (Table 16). Many composita preparations include suis-organ preparations. The organ to be targeted therapeutically is usually included as an 8X potency of the homologous suis-organ preparation, while other organs involved in the targeted physiological cycle are included as 10X potencies (e.g., Cutis compositum, Hepar compositum). For example, the preparation Hepar compositum includes the ingredient Hepar suis as an 8X potency, while Vesica fellea suis, Pancreas suis, Duodenum suis, Colon suis, and Thymus suis are included as 10X potencies.

Solidago compositum S (ampules)
Composition:
10 plant ingredients in the form of single potencies
Solidago 3X (goldenrod)
Berberis 4X (barberry)
Terebinthina 6X (turpentine)
Bucco 8X (bucco leaves)
Capsicum 6X (hot pepper)
Orthosiphon stamineus 6X (Java tea)
Equisetum hiemale 4X (common horsetail)
Pareira brava 6X
Baptisia 4X (false indigo)
Sarsaparilla 6X (sarsaparilla)
2 animal ingredients in the form of single potencies
Cantharis (Lytta vesicatoria) 6X (Spanish fly)
Apisinum 8X (bee venom)
5 mineral ingredients in the form of single potencies
Hydrargyrum bicloratum 8X (mercuric chloride)
Arsenicum album D28 (white arsenic)
Cuprum sulfuricum 6X (copper sulfate)
Hepar sulfuris 8X
Argentum nitricum 6X (silver nitrate)

> **4 potentized organ preparations in the form of single potencies**
>   Vesica urinaria suis 8X (bladder)
>   Pyelon suis 10X (renal pelvis)
>   Ureter suis 10X (ureter)
>   Urethra suis 10X (urethra)
> **3 nosodes in the form of single potencies**
>   Pyrogenium 198X
>   Colibacillinum 13X
>   Coxsackie-Virus A_9-Nosode 8X
> **1 intermediary catalyst in the form of a single potency**
>   Natrium pyruvicum 10X

Tab.16: Example of the composition of a "multifaceted" composita preparation with ingredients from different classes of substances

Intermediary catalysts (as in Coenzyme compositum, Causticum compositum), and/or homeopathically adjusted allopathic remedies (as in Echinacea compositum S), and/or nosodes may be included in composita preparations, either in addition to or instead of suis-organ preparations. A few composita preparations that may trigger massive release of toxins (such as Colchicum compositum and Viscum compositum, both used as adjunct therapies for neoplasms) are available in mite, medium, and forte forms, with the potency levels decreasing from the mite to the forte form (Table 17). The same applies to Echinacea compositum S, which is also available in a forte form.

Most composita preparations are available as ampules and/or drops. In individual instances, other forms such as tablets (Molybdän compositum), suppositories (Atropinum compositum), and nasal spray (Euphorbium compositum) are available.

Colchicum compositum mite S (ampules)
Composition:
5 plant ingredients in the form of single potencies
Colchicum 6X (colchicum)
Conium 4X (poison hemlock)
Galium aparine 4X (cleavers)
Podophyllum 4X (mayapple)
Hydrastis 4X (goldenseal)

Colchicum compositum medium S (ampules)
Composition:
5 plant ingredients in the form of single potencies
Colchicum 5X (colchicum)
Conium 3X (poison hemlock)
Galium aparine 3X (cleavers)
Podophyllum 3X (mayapple)
Hydrastis 3X (goldenseal)

Colchicum compositum forte S (ampules)
Composition:
5 plant ingredients in the form of single potencies
Colchicum 4X (colchicum)
Conium 2X (poison hemlock)
Galium aparine 2X (cleavers)
Podophyllum 2X (mayapple)
Hydrastis 3X (goldenseal)

Tab.17: Example of the composition of a composita preparation available in different strengths

4.3.2 Single-Constituent Homeopathic Preparations

Homeopathic single-constituent preparations may be used in antihomotoxic therapy. Use of a single-constituent preparation is recommended when its drug picture matches the patient's symptoms. Selection and therapeutic use is governed by the Law of Similars.

This category includes two distinctly different types of preparations: single-constituent preparations in potency chords (injeels) and single-constituent preparations in single potencies.

Injeels, along with combination preparations, play a central role in antihomotoxic injection therapy. Injeels, which are available in injectable form (ampules) and contain individual substances in the form of potency chords, are described in greater detail below.

Single-Constituent Preparations in Potency Chords (Injeels)

Preparations that are packed in ampules and contain single-constituent preparations in the form of potency chords are called injeels (*inj*ection + H*eel*). Most of the remedies of the homeopathic materia medica and all others belonging to the antihomotoxic repertory (homeopathically adjusted allopathic remedies, catalysts, nosodes, and suis-organ preparations) are available as injeels. Most injeels are available in both a simple and a forte form. The base potency in an injeel is usually 10X or 12X, with 30X and 200X added, while the corresponding injeel forte also includes a low potency, generally 4X or 6X. For more information, see the section on homaccords.

Single-Constituent Preparations in Single Potencies

In this group, medications intended for parenteral therapy are distinguished from those for oral therapy. Nosodes, catalysts, and homeopathically adjusted allopathic remedies, along with some of the classic homeopathic remedies in selected potency levels, are available as ready-to-use medications for parenteral administration as single-constituent preparations in single potencies.

Single potencies of any ingredient in antihomotoxic parenteral medications can be specially ordered in the form of dilutions and globules for oral administration. The other classes of medications used in homotoxicology (homeopathically adjusted allopathic remedies, catalysts, nosodes, and suis-organ preparations) are also available in liquid form as single substances in single potencies.

4.3.3 Homeopathically Adjusted Allopathic Remedies

This group of medications, introduced into therapeutic use by homotoxicology, includes a number of agents in common use in conventional medicine, especially antibiotics and antipyretics. These "allopathic" medications are further processed in accordance with the guidelines of the German homeopathic pharmacopoeia (HAB) and are available as potency chords packaged in ampules (injeels or injeels forte).

The use of these preparations is based on the concept that the reversal of effect caused by potentization allows a potentized allopathic medication to alleviate damage caused by allopathic doses of the same medication or to prevent such damage if the two medications are taken simultaneously. Furthermore, such preparations induce mobilization and elimination of remnants of previously ingested allopathic medications that have not yet been, or cannot be, removed. In this sense, homeopathically adjusted allopathic remedies could be called "foreign substance nosodes" in an analogy to classic nosodes. Like the latter, homeopathically adjusted allopathic remedies clear the biological terrain of the same substances or their sequelae and residues. This model is confirmed by the results of various experiments using dilutions of allopathic medications. (11, 32) The homeopathic dilution need not contain exactly the same active chemical compound that caused the damage; a related chemical will serve the same purpose. Doutremepuich reports on the effects of ultra-low doses of chemicals or medications. (8)

4.3.4 Intermediary Catalysts

Therapeutic use of catalysts involved in intermediary metabolism is unique to antihomotoxic therapy. The chemicals known as intermediary catalysts arise during and catalyze the processes of cellular respiration and energy metabolism (citric acid cycle, redox systems) and certain other enzymatic conversions. Because many conventional pharmaceuticals work by influencing enzymes, damage to enzyme systems is frequently of iatrogenic origin. Increases in environmental loading (e.g., heavy metals, pesticides, electromagnetic pollution) further compromise enzyme functions. Failure of an enzyme function causes accumulation of metabolites produced in earlier reactions and deficiencies of metabolites that would be formed in subsequent reactions.

The purpose of administering homeopathic doses of appropriate catalysts is to activate metabolic processes and restore blocked cellular and enzymatic functions. This class of medications is especially suited to treating the chronic or degenerative diseases that are the chief manifestations of enzyme damage.

The preparations available can be divided into three groups:

▶ **Group A: acids of the citric acid cycle**
Metabolites of carbohydrates, fats, and proteins all feed into the citric acid cycle, the metabolism's central hub. In conjunction with the respiratory chain, the citric acid cycle provides the prerequisites for ATP formation and thus for the release of energy for metabolic reactions.

▶ **Group B: quinones, quinone derivatives, and other intermediary respiratory catalysts**
The primary reactive group in these compounds is the carbonyl group. Depolymerization by the carbonyl group blocks condensation processes in the body, which occur during the phases of impregnation, degeneration, and especially dedifferentiation. Viral toxins, damage due to immunization or antibiotics, and autointoxication originating in the intestines can all trigger occupation of the carbonyl group of the respiratory enzyme by amines. Quinones and other carbonyl-containing compounds break these bonds and restore the function of the original carbonyl group through oxidative radical reaction mechanisms. (14) Koch provides more detailed information on this process. (19)

▶ **Group C: other compounds with stimulant effects**
This group includes homeopathic preparations of various compounds such as hormones, vitamins, biogenic amines, trace elements (cerium), and plant extracts (anthocyanins)

Table 18 gives examples of these three groups of catalyst preparations.

Antihomotoxic Biotherapeutic Medications

All intermediary catalysts are available as single-constituent preparations in potency chords (see the section on injeels and injeels forte), and some are available in single potencies. They also are included in many composita preparations, Coenzyme compositum and Ubichinon compositum in particular.

1. Group A – potentized acids of the citric acid cycle
Examples:
Acidum cis-aconiticum-Injeel (forte)
Acidum citricum-Injeel (forte)
Acidum fumaricum-Injeel (forte)
Acidum α-ketoglutaricum-Injeel (forte)
Acidum DL-malicum-Injeel (forte)
Natrium oxalaceticum-Injeel (forte)
Natrium pyruvicum-Injeel (forte)

2. Group B – potentized quinones and other intermediary respiratory catalysts
Examples:
Anthrachinon-Injeel (forte)
Para-Benzochinon-Injeel (forte)
Hydrochinon-Injeel (forte)
Methylglyoxal-Injeel (forte)
Methylenblau-Injeel (forte)
Ubichinon-Injeel (forte)

3. Group C - homeopathic preparations of other compounds that stimulate metabolic functions
Examples:
Acidum L(+)-asparagicum-Injeel (forte)
Acidum L(+)-lacticum-Injeel (forte)
Cerium oxalicum-Injeel (forte)
Cystein-Injeel (forte)
Scatol-Injeel (forte)
Vitamin A-Injeel (forte)
Vitamin B_6-Injeel (forte)

Tab.18: Examples of different groups of intermediary catalyst preparations

4.3.5 Nosodes

As defined in the German homeopathic pharmacopoeia (HAB), nosodes are medications produced homeopathically from pathologically altered human organs (or parts of organs), killed cultures of microorganisms, breakdown products of animal organs, or body fluids that no longer contain virulent or infectious pathogens or by-products of disease (see HAB 1, general instructions and rules 43, 44, and AMG §3, section 3 and 4).

The first step in the production of nosodes under HAB guidelines is sterilization of the raw material, followed by testing for sterility in accordance with the German pharmacopoeia (DAB 10). Because potentization takes place only after sterility has been guaranteed, nosodes are not vaccines or serums and monitoring by the Paul Ehrlich Institute of the Bundesgesundheitsamt (German Federal Department of Public Health) is not required.

Therapy with nosodes is based on the concept that homeopathic potencies of by-products of disease stimulate specific immune responses. According to Mezger, (23) nosodes can be used in three ways:

▶ As isotherapy, i.e., a nosode can be administered as specific therapy for the disease from which it is derived. In such cases the nosode is administered alternately with indicated homeopathic remedies.

▶ As homeotherapy (i.e., according to the Law of Similars). Drug pictures for some nosodes have been determined through drug testing, experience in their therapeutic use, and observation of the corresponding illnesses (e.g., Tuberculinum, Medorrhinum, Luesinum, Psorinum).

▶ As a drainage remedy. After recovery from an illness, nosodes are an excellent means of eliminating toxins deposited in the mesenchyme. "Such cases often require the elimination not only of germ toxins but also of germ remnants with latent disease foci and germ colonies that are no longer pathogenic (as in permanent carriers)." (23) For this reason, nosodes have often been called "biological terrain remedies."

Table 19 categorizes the use of nosodes in terms of different levels of similarity.

1. Symptomatic similarity (i.e., according to the Law of Similars)
2. Prior etiological (anamnestisch-ätiologisch) similarity (illnesses in the patient's earlier medical history that seem to have been cured)
3. Current etiological similarity (at the beginning of an acute illness)
4. Recent etiological similarity (at the end of an illness)
5. Desensitization

Tab.19: Levels of similarity in nosode therapy (1, 9, 18)

Some authors with experience in veterinary medicine have demonstrated that prophylactic administration of a nosode prepared from either pathognomonic pathogens or affected organs seems to confer protection against contracting the disease in question. (20, 37)

At this point we must mention briefly the issue of drug safety as it applies to nosodes. We cannot simply assume that medications such as nosodes, which are derived from pathologically damaged or infectious raw materials, are harmless. Empirical studies in human and veterinary medicine on the issue of nosode safety report no evidence of adverse effects. Gratz administered various nosodes to many pets in her small-animal veterinary practice without observing any adverse effects. (15) A prospective study conducted by Werthmann on the administration of nosodes gathered data on 188 patients; responses to the questionnaires contained no reports of adverse effects. (39)

The safety of nosode preparations also has been tested in experimental studies conducted under laboratory conditions. At the Public Health Institute of the University of Heidelberg, 25 different nosodes in low potencies were tested for sterility and for the presence of endotoxins and pathogenicity factors (coagulase, streptokinase). With a single exception (one low-potency preparation contained barely detectable levels of endotoxins), all findings were negative, even with regard to nosodes manufactured from gram-negative bacteria. This study also concluded that the combination of sterilization and homeopathic dilution rendered the active substances nonallergenic and that administering such homeopathic preparations entails "an extremely low level of risk."(31)

Experiments conducted by the Battelle Institute used sinusitis nosode as a model for determining whether the infectivity-reducing measures integrated into standard nosode production methods (which are the same regardless of the raw material) effectively inactivate microorganisms. (5) Test pathogens added to the samples included vaccinia and polio viruses, a bacterium (*Bacillus stearothermophilus*), and a fungus (*Aspergillus niger*). Standardized production methods were then applied to the infected preparations. Postproduction testing demonstrated that all of the test microorganisms were completely inactivated.

In summary, the safety of nosode preparations has been thoroughly established, both in practice and through experimental studies. Additional information on drug safety and issues of risk can be found in the chapter on suis-organ preparations (p. 71 ff.).

In homotoxicology, nosodes are used primarily to induce reversion of cellular phases to humoral phases, but they also may be administered in humoral phases when the illness threatens to become chronic. The use of nosodes in acute phases of illness may provoke excessive reactions and therefore must be administered with caution.

Like the catalysts and homeopathically adjusted allopathic remedies, nosodes are available as individual substances in the form of potency chords (injeels and injeels forte, see p. 62 ff.), and some are available in single potencies. They also are included in some of the composita preparations.

Several different systems for classifying nosodes have been proposed. Julian distinguishes pure microbial cultures from products defined in the pharmacopoeia and from by-products of disease taken directly from the patient. Alternatively, he distinguishes between basic and diathetic nosodes, further subdividing the latter into psoriatic, sycotic, tubercular, luetic, and isopathic groups. (18) In homotoxicology, antihomotoxic nosode preparations are classified as followed:

▶ Pathogenic nosodes: When a medically definable pathogen substrate (such as *Streptococcus* or *Escherichia coli*
bacteria), -Injeel is added to the name of the pathogen to
form the name of the medication (e.g., Streptococcus-In-
jeel).

▶ Tissue nosodes: When a discharge is reliably associated
with a specific illness, or in the case of preparations derived from pathologically altered tissue, -Nosode-Injeel
is added to the name of the illness (e.g., Sinusitis-
Nosode-Injeel).

▶ Other substances of biological origin that often are considered allergenic (such as eggs, milk, and fat) are also
potentized for use in antihomotoxic therapy. For histori-
cal reasons, these preparations are also called nosodes
even though they do not fit the definition given above,
and -Injeel is added to the name of the substance in
question.

Table 20 gives examples of nosode preparations.

1. **Pathogen nosodes**: suspensions of pathogens raised
   in pure cultures, killed by sterilization and homeopathi-
   cally potentized
   Examples:
   Ascariden-Injeel (forte)
   Arthritis urica-Nosode-Injeel (forte)
   Bacterium proteus-Injeel (forte)
   Bacterium pyocyaneus-Injeel (forte)
   Coxsackie-Virus A_9-Injeel (forte)
   Diphtherinum-Injeel (forte)
   Klebsiella pneumoniae-Injeel (forte)
   Pertussis-Nosode-Injeel (forte)
   Staphylococcus-Injeel (forte)
   Streptococcus haemolyticus-Injeel (forte)

2. **Tissue nosodes**: preparations derived from diseased organs or tissues, inactivated by sterilization, and homeopathically potentized
Examples:
Adenoma mammae-Injeel (forte)
Appendicitis-Nosode-Injeel (forte)
Calculi renales-Injeel (forte)
Carcinoma bronchium-Injeel (forte)
Cirrhosis hepatis-Nosode-Injeel (forte)
Granuloma dentis-Injeel (forte)
Hepatitis-Nosode-Injeel (forte)
Meningeoma-Injeel (forte)
Parodontose-Nosode-Injeel (forte)
Struma parenchymatosa-Injeel (forte)

3. **Other preparations also called nosodes**: homeopathic potencies of other substances of biological origin that are used in antihomotoxic stimulation therapy
Examples:
Adeps suillus-Injeel (forte)
Cerumen-Injeel
Crinis humanus-Injeel (forte)
Fel tauri-Injeel (forte)
Lac caninum-Injeel (forte)
Ovum Injeel (forte)
Serum ovile-Injeel (forte)

Tab. 20: Classification of nosodes according to the substances from which they are derived

4.3.6 Suis-Organ Preparations

Preparations derived from animal organs are used both in antihomotoxic therapy and in anthroposophical medicine. The suis-organ preparations used in homotoxicology, which are homeopathically prepared in accordance with HAB guidelines, are made from organ tissues taken from healthy hogs raised under carefully monitored conditions. At the end of the production process, the ampules are sterilized according to HAB 1, Regulation 11, as required by DAB 10. Because sterilization is the final step, qualitative aspects of the living tissue are preserved during potentization, and the protein in the preparations relates directly to the patient's diseased organs. The oral forms of these preparations are not sterilized but are subjected to postproduction microbiological testing. Results must meet DAB 10 standards.

The hog was chosen as the donor animal because it is very similar to the human organism in many characteristics such as tissue structure, metabolism, biochemistry, and susceptibility to specific infections and vascular diseases. Thus, hog tissues can be considered a simile of human tissues. The working mechanism of a suis-organ preparation is based on affinity between the patient's diseased organ and that from which the medication is derived. In fresh cell therapy (which is based on a similar principle but implemented with materially present rather than potentized quantities of substrate), radiolabeling has demonstrated that when cells or cell fragments are administered, they are drawn to the related organ (organotropism); that is, organ similarity outweighs the difference in species. (13) However, suis-organ therapy, which involves totally different production methods and quantities of substances that are smaller by several powers of 10, should not be confused with either fresh cell therapy or treatment with organotherapeutics.

Regarding drug safety, in a deposition by a scientific expert witness, Schmid distinguishes three different areas of theoretical risk with regard to potentized organ preparations. (30) Schmid states that organ preparations from healthy mammalian donor animals, such as those from whom the raw materials for suis-organ preparations are derived, are harmless from the toxicological perspective. Even when the raw materials are enzymatically active tissues (e.g., Duodenum suis) or tissues colonized by bacteria (Colon suis), all evidence of endotoxins disappears at a 4X level of dilution. Schmid notes that concentrations of active substances in the 2X to 5X range can be used in allergic desensitization and that although substances at these dilution levels may provoke local reactions, no serious immunological reactions should occur. At potencies of 6X and higher, there is no longer even a theoretical risk of allergic reactions. With regard to the possibility of infection, Schmid found no evidence that the undiluted mother tinctures supported the growth of various pathogenic bacteria and viruses with which they were inoculated.

So-called unconventional viruses are of greatest concern with regard to the possibility of direct viral infection, but to date no spontaneous cases of spongiform encephalopathy have been observed in hogs. Worldwide, only one hog has been successfully infected with the disease in deliberate attempts under the strictest laboratory conditions. (6) Schmid points out that to date only 11 cases of subacute spongiform encephalopathy in humans have been associated with therapeutic use of human organ tissues. The cases in question involved human growth hormone, dura mater, and a cornea transplant. (30) Although animal organ preparations have been used for decades, there is still no evidence that they transmit animal-specific viruses to humans.

Straub determined that no viruses or bacteria endemic to hogs survive heat sterilization of the suis-organ preparations intended for parenteral administration. (36)

Studies have been conducted to determine the allergenic potential of ready-to-use medications containing suis-organ preparations. (34) Immune diffusion experiments used a hog antiserum in an attempt to demonstrate the presence of hog proteins in the combination preparation Zeel P but found none after the autoclaving typical of the production process. In a second experiment, guinea pigs were sensitized to the hog protein used in the production of Zeel P. Intradermal reexposure to the antigen at a dilution of 1:20000 triggered positive skin reactions, but a challenge application of the ready-to-use medication, which contains a 1:108 dilution of hog tissue extract, provoked no allergic reactions in the test animals. (34)

In conclusion, the combination of many measures that reduce infectivity or eliminate the possibility of infection (monitoring and selection of donor animals and breeding stock, use of tissues or organs with low theoretical risk potentials, production measures such as autoclaving and homeopathic dilution, methods of administration, and the existence of a species barrier) renders suis-organ preparations harmless and guarantees that "the oft-cited potential risk to the patient being treated is more of a matter of theoretical speculation than an near-reality." (30)

With regard to their therapeutic effects, suis-organ preparations extend the scope of the classic homeopathic repertory to include the treatment of organ dysfunctions and degenerative organ damage. In antihomotoxic therapy, therefore, suis-organ preparations are used primarily to stimulate specific organs in phases to the right of the biological division. Immunological responses may be responsible for the efficacy of these preparations.

Single suis-organ preparations are available as potency chords (injeels and injeels forte) and are most frequently administered in these forms. They also are included in many composita preparations. The selection of the organ or tissue and the potencies in the composita preparations have been discussed. Combining the organ preparations with other homeopathic ingredients seems to help them target the appropriate organ more effectively. According to the clinical experiences of various authors, suis-organ preparations also enhance the efficacy of the other ingredients.

4.4 Administering and Combining Antihomotoxic Ampule Preparations

Many practitioners have observed that simultaneous treatment with several antihomotoxic medications is often useful, especially in cases of chronic illness. The results of therapy are often better when remedies are combined than when a single medication is administered.

To date no chemical or physical-energetic interactions have been observed when preparations diluted to levels of 4X or higher are combined in mixed injections, and no intolerance symptoms have been documented in conjunction with the use of injected combinations. Thus, multiple antihomotoxic remedies can be administered parenterally either as individual injections or as a single mixed injection.

Ampule preparations may be administered orally. The ampules are emptied into a small glass of water, which the patient drinks one sip at a time over the course of the day. To take advantage of absorption via the oral mucosa, the liquid should be held in the mouth for a while before it is swallowed.

5. The Therapeutic Use of Antihomotoxic Medications

Having described the different classes of medications used in antihomotoxic therapy, we will now explain how these preparations are used in the context of a total treatment plan.

Unless the practitioner is already familiar with the patient's medical history, a detailed case history should be compiled before therapy is begun. It should include both the patient's current health status as well as all earlier illnesses and their treatment. In many respects, a thorough case history provides important information with regard to which specific antihomotoxic medications can be expected to produce good results.

The following factors are especially important in selecting individually appropriate antihomotoxic medications:

▶ the patient's current symptoms
▶ acute or chronic status of the current illness
▶ any prior illnesses and treatments reported by the patient.

What information do the patient's symptoms provide with regard to selecting an antihomotoxic medication? In classical homeopathy the selection of an individually appropriate remedy that matches the patient's symptoms is made according to Hahnemann. This truism has often led to the erroneous conclusion that homeopathy attempts to treat symptoms, while in fact understanding the patient's symptoms in detail is merely an aid to finding a remedy that effectively targets the underlying illness. According to Reckeweg's homotoxin theory, the patient's symptoms are indicators of the types of toxins that the diseased organism's immune system must tackle. Reckeweg says, "Each toxic status presents a typical set of symptoms that expedites the search for an effective antihomotoxic agent." (24) Consequently, administering a trace amount of a toxin or a medication provides a subtle stimulus that mobilizes additional endogenous defense forces against the toxins causing the immediate illness. Patient-specific medications are selected according to the Law of Similars, similia similibus curentur, "likes may be cured by likes." Thus, Reckeweg's homotoxin theory also sheds light on why a low dose may effectively treat the very symptoms that a higher dose of the same substance provokes in healthy individuals.

In general terms, homotoxicology defines disease processes as manifestations of either toxin damage or the body's defensive measures against toxins. However, this does not mean that every illness is caused by a single, clearly defined homotoxin. In most cases behind each diagnosed illness stands a relatively complex event involving the simultaneous effects of a number of different toxins on different tissues. The complexity of most disease processes requires a multifaceted approach to therapy. In addition to avoiding the introduction of additional homotoxins, such an approach also involves administering specific antihomotoxic combination medications whose ingredients provide broad support for the body's various levels of defense.

Reckeweg made a comprehensive assortment of homeopathic combination remedies for antihomotoxic therapy. Because the range of therapeutic effects of each combination medication targets a specific syndrome, these preparations generally can be prescribed according to clinical diagnoses, which not only simplifies the therapeutic use of homeopathic medications considerably but also permits homeopathic treatment of illnesses whose symptoms do not correspond to the drug pictures of any of the classical homeopathic remedies.

Reckeweg himself often used homeopathic single remedies (usually in the form of injeels or injeels forte) when the patient's symptoms reflected a clearly recognizable drug picture. He also observed that many patients, especially at the very beginning of treatment, present constellations of symptoms that do not correspond to any single drug picture, a phenomenon he interpreted as meaning that at this stage the diseased body is beset by many toxins at once, and their effects overlap to such an extent that it is impossible to recognize a single clear drug picture. In such cases Reckeweg recommended administering several combination remedies to address all the patient's symptoms simultaneously. For example, medications for headache, cardiac symptoms, venostasis, and joint pain could be administered together. Even when the patient presents constellations of symptoms in which many different drug pictures overlap, making it impossible to prescribe a classical homeopathic remedy, the broad spectrum of activity of the antihomotoxic combination preparations guarantees activation of specific defense mechanisms to counteract the homotoxins involved in the illness.

Reckeweg recommends "covering the entire complex of symptoms with suitable antihomotoxics" and "utilizing multiple prescriptions in cases involving multiple toxins." (24) Symptoms often change as newly strengthened defensive functions eliminate individual homotoxins. Some symptoms may recede or disappear while others move to the foreground. Leimbach describes this process as "gradually unearthing the homotoxins," just as a buried monument is gradually exposed during an archeological dig. (29) As treatment progresses and many homotoxins are bound and eliminated, symptoms corresponding to a typical drug picture often emerge. This may be a sign that the homotoxins have been largely eliminated; as a rule, a single remedy is then sufficient to eliminate the remaining toxins and facilitate the patient's complete recovery. Reckeweg says, "The toxins may have to be encircled by a whole regiment that is, one or more combination preparations and additional units may need to be drawn into the detoxification battle before the last remaining basic homotoxin, the 'commander of the enemy forces', can be finished off with the single pistol shot of the similimum." (29)

5.1. The Influence of Acute or Chronic Status on Therapy

5.1.1 Acute Illnesses

In developing an individual treatment plan, not only the symptoms but also the acute or chronic status of an illness also must be considered. From the perspective of homotoxin theory, inflammation and other acute symptoms usually indicate that the patient is in the inflammation phase, i.e., the diseased organism's defense systems are heavily involved in attempting to control the homotoxic loading. The homeopathic remedies of the classical materia medica, either as single remedies or combination preparations, are generally effective in treating acute illnesses. The basic principle is that acute disease states require low potencies (such as the forte form of the injeels) and frequent administration of indicated remedies (Table 21). The more severe and acute the symptoms, the more frequently the remedies should be administered.

For initial treatment of acute cases, medications in tablet and drop form can be administered at a dosage of one tablet or ten drops every 15 minutes for up to two hours, while injectables are generally administered once a day but may be given up to three times a day in exceptional cases. Careful observation of the patient's progress is important during massive-dose therapy. The frequency of the doses should be reduced gradually as soon as improvement in symptoms is noted. If the patient's symptoms worsen, it may be necessary to discontinue the massive-dose therapy and introduce a different medication. Individual circumstances alone can determine the course to take.

Status of illness	Acute illness	Chronic Illness
Type of antihomotoxic medication to be administered	In most cases, potentized substances from the classical materia medica (either as single remedies or in combination preparations)	Classical homeopathic remedies in combination with intermediary catalysts, potentized allopathic drugs, nosodes, or suis-organ preparations
Potency levels of the medications administered	Low potencies (< D6)	High and very high potencies
Dosage of antihomotoxic medications	Frequent administration of the indicated remedies (as massive-dose therapy, if needed)	Less frequent doses of the indicated medications

Tab. 21: Antihomotoxic therapy for acute and chronic disease states

5.1.2 Chronic Diseases

As a rule, chronic disease states require a different therapeutic strategy. From the homotoxicological perspective, chronically ill patients are already in either the deposition phase or one of the phases to the right of the biological division (impregnation, degeneration, or dedifferentiation). Any chronic illness indicates either that the patient's defense systems cannot cope with the constant or recurrent presence of homotoxins or that endogenous defenses against noxae have been damaged or hindered by attacks from outside, such as inappropriate therapeutic measures. As a general rule, the massive homotoxin loading and weakened immune status typical of chronic illness make it inadvisable to intervene with low potencies (i.e., overly high concentrations) or overly frequent doses of homeopathic remedies, for fear of exacerbating the homotoxin situation.

In chronic cases, therefore, indicated medications are not administered in the form of massive-dose therapy but rather in standard doses of one tablet or ten drops three times a day or, in the case of injectables (which may also be administered as mixed injections), one ampule one to three times a week. If the correct medications are selected, the relatively "gentle" stimuli provided by the standard dosage are often enough to gradually reactivate the body's defense systems.

In chronic conditions, however, the substances of the classical homeopathic materia medica, if used alone, are often insufficient to normalize the body's disturbed detoxification functions. Physiological disturbances or damage to cellular structures accompany many chronic illnesses, especially those homotoxicology describes as belonging to phases to the right of the biological division (impregnation, degeneration, and dedifferentiation). This insight prompted Reckeweg to supplement classical homeopathic therapy with the class of substances that he called intermediary catalysts, homeopathic preparations of chemicals recognized by biochemistry as essential to the physiological processes of human metabolism. Administering these substances in very high potencies provides subtle stimuli intended to reactivate metabolic processes and restore blocked cellular and enzymatic functions. Homeopathic remedies derived from organs, such as the suis-organ preparations, also often improve the functioning of cellular structures. These of homeopathic medications offer the possibilty of successful treatment for chronic illnesses, even those of long duration.

5.2 The Importance of Prior Illnesses for Therapy

In developing an antihomotoxic treatment, the patient's entire medical history, including any therapy for prior illnesses, should be considered. According to homotoxin theory, a patient's illnesses are usually vicariating phases of a single homotoxicosis rather than isolated phenomena. Reckeweg says, "When eczema patients begin to suffer asthma attacks after their skin problems have been resolved through conventional therapy and when they then have to accept eczema again in exchange for freedom from the asthma, vicariation phenomena are at work." (27) According to Reckeweg's theory, seemingly unrelated illnesses may be caused by the same homotoxin as it shifts from one tissue to another, provoking different responses, i.e., different symptoms.

The patient's prior illnesses are significant with regard to current therapy in two respects. First, toxin-specific endogenous defenses are stimulated when either a homeopathic single remedy chosen according to the simile principle or an indication-specific antihomotoxic combination remedy is administered. This process may cause the illness-triggering homotoxins to shift to a different tissue, where they may provoke flare-ups of supposedly eradicated symptoms while the patient's current symptoms improve. Such flare-ups often involve inflammations of the skin or of the nose and throat mucosae (eczema, rhinitis, pharyngitis, peritonsilar abscesses, etc.).

Second, responses to antihomotoxic medications often also include escalated elimination processes, whether physiological (e.g., increased urination) or seemingly pathological (e.g., leukorrhea, formation of fistulas). Reckeweg sees such processes as prognostically favorable regressive vicariations that indicate that the organism is actively grappling with the disease-triggering homotoxins. Quite understandably, however, the patient experiences such reactions as impediments to well-being. Therefore, before beginning therapy it is advisable to counsel the patient on these predictable indispositions and the context in which they occur so that they will not be interpreted as new symptoms or adverse effects of the antihomotoxic medication. Because patients are increasingly critical of the risks of drug therapy, it is important to distinguish adverse effects from reactions that serve a biological purpose in the healing process. Reckeweg's Six-Phase table can be very helpful, because if the symptoms that reappear during antihomotoxic therapy fall further up or to the left on the table than the patient's primary illness, it is safe to assume that a prognostically favorable regressive vicariation has occurred. Admittedly, proper classification of all possible initial reactions requires a certain amount of therapeutic experience. Dealing with such phenomena, however, is very important in the practice of antihomotoxic therapy, not only because skillfully explaining vicariation symptoms in context can encourage patient compliance but also because the practitioner gains added confidence in developing treatment plans.

5.3 Options for Treating Problematic Cases

In many patients, residual homotoxic damage due to earlier illnesses or their treatment is so serious that classical homeopathic remedies alone are not enough to permanently rectify the toxic situation. When high doses of synthetic chemical drugs are taken repeatedly or for extended periods, homotoxic loading often occurs as a result of the drugs themselves. In such cases, however, administering homeopathic dilutions of the same substance or a similar one often reverses damage triggered by the effects of allopathic medications. It is always very important to question the patient about treatment for prior illnesses because administering the appropriate homeopathic potencies of allopathic drugs often achieves decisive breakthroughs in cases of chronic illness.

In other instances, when the functions of specific organs or cells have been damaged as a direct result of pathogen toxins, nosodes often perform well as "biological terrain remedies." A trial of nosode therapy is indicated if the patient has ever experienced the appearance of new symptoms in connection with an infection or if there is even a chance that current symptoms are related to incomplete recovery from an earlier illness.

5.4 Bioelectronic Testing

Although experienced practitioners who are aware of the issues raised here and familiar with available medications can select the most individually appropriate antihomotoxic therapy with a great degree of certainty, many practitioners also successfully use bioelectronic techniques for selecting medications (Electroacupuncture (EAV) according to Voll, other methods of bioelectronic testing). It must be emphasized, however, that bioelectronic methods are not indispensable to antihomotoxic therapy but simply aid in determining the most effective medication in an individual case. Bioelectronic techniques are not unique to homotoxicology and can be used equally well in conjunction with other types of therapy.

Although the testing techniques listed above can also be used for diagnostic purposes, they are no substitute for regular medical diagnosis. Their particular strength lies in discovering bioenergetic regulatory disturbances. In contrast, they are of very limited value in confirming or eliminating the possibility of pathological anatomical changes.

Various manufacturers produce equipment used for taking bioelectronic readings. Such equipment generally consists of a probe, an inert hand-held electrode, a honeycomb grid to hold sample vials, and the actual measuring device itself. Electroacupuncture according to Voll will be described briefly as an example of such procedures. This method is based on the assumption that readings of skin resistance at acupuncture points associated with specific organs reflect the physiological status of these organs. To take a skin resistance reading, a probe is pressed lightly against the skin at precise points and the score registers on a scale divided into 100 units. Readings in the 40 to 60 range are considered normal, while lower or higher readings indicate pathological processes. Downward movement of the pointer as the reading is being taken is an additional indicator of pathological change in the organ in question. After many practitioners observed that the reading often changed when the patient takes a medication in his/her hand, the possibility of using this method to test medications was investigated further. The procedure has been adapted to include a honeycomb grid that is wired into the test circuit and holds vials of medications. Based on years of experience on the part of many practitioners, we can expect positive effects from medications that increase the score.

Test kits that include all available preparations in each class of antihomotoxic medications (e.g., nosodes, potentized allopathic drugs, suis-organ preparations) have become available in recent years to aid systematic testing of medications. As a result, the process of determining individually appropriate antihomotoxic medications has become significantly easier.

5.5 Graduated Auto-Sanguis Therapy

Graduated auto-sanguis therapy is a variant of autohemotherapy that differs from the standard form in that it potentizes the patient's own blood for use as an autonosode. This therapy has proved very effective in treating a variety of chronic or degenerative disorders such as bronchial asthma, eczema, liver damage, and many others. According to Reckeweg's homotoxin theory, almost all diseases can be defined as manifestations of either toxin-induced damage or the organism's defensive responses to toxins. Presumably, then, each patient's blood contains pathognomonic homotoxins. According to Reckeweg, removing small amounts of blood and reinjecting it into the body after potentizing it to several different levels uses these specific toxins as isotherapeutic stimulants. According to the Arndt-Schulz Law, the effects of low concentrations of substances are the opposite of those of high concentrations.[1] Consequently, the potentized, individually specific toxins used in auto-sanguis therapy promote healing by stimulating increased detoxification activity by endogenous defense systems. The addition of individually appropriate homeopathic injectables further enhances the effect of the patient's own potentized blood, as per Bürgi's Principle,[2] so the practice of using ampule preparations as the medium for potentizing the patient's blood has proved expedient. Presumably, auto-sanguis therapy supports natural recovery by counteracting not only exogenous but also endogenous homotoxins such as toxic by-products of cell breakdown.

In practice, graduated auto-sanguis therapy is implemented as follows. A hypodermic syringe is used to withdraw blood from a vein and is then emptied until only tiny amounts of blood remain in the conical tip. For the first stage of auto-sanguis therapy, an indicated injeel, suis-organ preparation, potentized allopathic drug, or similar medication or medications (generally one, two, or more ampules) is drawn into the syringe, leaving a little empty space so that mixing occurs when the syringe is shaken. (The needle should be capped before shaking to prevent the liquid from escaping.) The syringe is shaken vigorously for approximately 10 strokes in the equivalent of the homeopathic process of potentization. The first dilution is then administered by intramuscular or subcutaneous injection, this time ejecting as much liquid as possible before reusing the same syringe. Only traces of the old injection solution should remain. After the syringe is again filled in the second stage with one or more ampules of a suitable preparation or preparations and shaken vigorously for 10 strokes, its contents are administered intramuscularly, subcutaneously, or intracutaneously. By repeating the process, a third, fourth, and even fifth stage can be implemented if necessary. The final stage can be injected intravenously. As a general rule, all five levels are administered in a single session.

In the process of producing the individual dilution levels, both the patient's blood and the preparations drawn into the syringe are homeopathically potentized and thus transformed into toxin-specific agents that stimulate increased detoxification by endogenous defensive mechanisms. It has also been suggested that the progressively diluted complement that is injected along with the patient's blood in graduated auto-sanguis therapy may have a homeopathic reversal effect on autoantibodies and antigen-antibody reactions. This phenomenon would explain the frequently observed positive effects of auto-sanguis therapy on autoimmune disorders. (10)

---

[1] Arndt-Schultz law: Vital functions are stimulated by weak impulses, promoted by moderately strong stimuli, inhibited by strong stimuli, and suspended by the very strongest stimuli.

[2] Bürgi's Principle: The effect of a combination of two different pharmaceuticals with equal or similar effects but different modes of action is not the sum of their separate effects. Instead, their efficacy is increased or potentized.

6. The Scientific Basis of Antihomotoxic Therapy

In conventional medical circles, complementary medicine is frequently criticized for the supposedly unscientific basis of the medications and therapeutic methods it espouses. However, such a sweeping generalization about all pharmaceutical companies in this category violates one of the first principles of scientific inquiry, namely, to be willing to thoroughly analyze each phenomenon while avoiding all bias or dogma.

This brief chapter aims to highlight the special position occupied by the Heel laboratories in the world of complementary medicine and to explain the scientific evidence that supports the Heel medications and methods of treatment. In this respect, the Heel laboratories compare favorably to pharmaceutical facilities in the allopathic sector. Heel's annual budget for scientific research amounts to one million dollar. This money is used to develop new medications, to study and improve the therapeutic efficacy of existing medications, and to make the results available to the medical profession through publications, instructional videos, and a scientific department that serves as a clearinghouse for expert information.

In addition to guaranteeing pure, high-quality medications that are produced to exacting specifications and packaged in appropriate doses, Heel's laboratory and field research provides incontestable proof of the therapeutic efficacy of Heel products, which meet the most stringent standards of pharmaceutical manufacturing (GMP, Good Manufacturing Practices).

6.1 Scientific Documentation

Heel biotherapeutic medications have been the subject of different types of scientific research, chiefly double- and single-blind studies, in vitro experiments, and market observation or monitoring studies. The list below, which presents several examples of publications for each type of study, includes only studies conducted on human subjects, although numerous animal studies also demonstrate the exceptional therapeutic efficacy of the most important Heel biotherapeutics. The animal studies, however, which eliminate the possibility of any placebo effects or suggestion, are actually even more interesting, since any observed therapeutic results can be attributed only to the medication itself.

6.1.1 Double-Blind Studies

Although double-blind studies generally confirm the therapeutic efficacy of the drugs being investigated, in the long run health care expenditures continue to increase rather than fall, despite repeated use of such drugs. Consequently, the value of this form of research has recently been called into question. Heel, however, has also profited from such research in the past. Several fascinating double-blind studies, two of which are listed below, compared a biotherapeutic preparation to an allopathic "best seller" used to treat the same symptoms. The results were surprising.

• Weiser M, Gegenheimer LH, Klein P. 1999. A randomized equivalence trial comparing the efficacy and safety of **Luffa compositum–Heel nasal spray** with cromolyn sodium spray in the treatment of seasonal allergic rhinitis. *Forschende Komplementärmedizin,* Vol. 6, No. 3. Comparative double-blind study of 146 patients with hay fever. Luffa compositum–Heel is as effective and well tolerated as cromolyn sodium. [E 117]

• Weiser M, Strösser W, Klein P. 1998. Homeopathic versus conventional treatment of vertigo. *Archives of Otolaryngology–Head & Neck Surgery,* Vol. 124, No. 8:879-885. Randomized double-blind study of 119 patients comparing **Vertigoheel®** to betahistine. Reduction in the frequency, duration, and severity of vertigo attacks was statistically significant with both forms of therapy. [E 115]

Other double-blind studies comparing biotherapeutics to placebos:

• Matusiewicz R. 1995. Efficacy of Engystol® N in asthma patients treated with corticosteroids. Double-blind study of 40 patients. During therapy with **Engystol® N**, clear improvement in symptoms is observed and corticosteroid dosage can be decreased. *Biological Therapy* 1995, No. 3:70–74 [1028]

• Weiser M, Clasen BPE. 1995. Treatment of chronic sinusitis with **Euphorbium compositum-nasal spray** versus placebo. Double-blind study of 155 patients. Euphorbium compositum-nasal spray is significantly more effective than placebo. *Biological Therapy,* Vol. 13, No. 1:4-11 [E 112]

• Böhmer D, Ambrus P (Frankfurt/Main University). 1992. Treatment of sports injuries with **Traumeel® S** ointment. Double-blind study of 102 patients. Evaluation criteria: maximum muscle strength, pain, swelling (circumference), and local skin temperature. **Traumeel®** S ointment was rated significantly more effective in all criteria. *Biological Therapy* 1992, No. 4:290-300 [E 97]

• Heilmann A. 1992. **Engystol® N** as a prophylactic in influenza. Double-blind study of 102 healthy males. Engystol® N delays (reduces) susceptibility to influenza. Symptoms disappeared significantly faster in prophylactically treated individuals. *Biological Therapy* 1994, No. 4:249-253 [E 108]

• Hamalcik P. 1994. Efficacy of **Euphorbium compositum-nasal spray S** versus physiological saline solution in chronic sinusitis. Double-blind study of 155 patients. Euphorbium compositum-nasal spray S is significantly more effective. *Biologische Medizin* 1994, Vol. 24, No. 1 [1018]

• Dietz A-R. 2000. Study of lymph therapy as matrix therapy for diabetic polyneuropathy in type II diabetics. Double-blind study of 90 patients, Lymphomyosot® versus α-lipoic acid. **Lymphomyosot®** reduces edema and is superior to conventional treatment in improving sensitivity and reducing pain. *Biologische Medizin* 2000, Vol.29, No. 1:4–9 [E 123]

6.1.2 Single-Blind Studies

Most of these studies compare a Heel preparation with a commercially available alternative. In the third example, the use of experimental animals also allows therapeutic efficacy to be confirmed according to objective standards.

• Nahler G. 1996. **Zeel® comp.** in osteoarthritis of the knee. Single-blind study of 114 patients comparing Zeel® comp. injections to Hyalart, a common German antirheumatic based on hyaluronic acid. The two medications were equally effective, but Zeel® comp. had 50% fewer adverse effects. *Orthopädische Praxis* Vol. 32, No. 5. *Biological Therapy* 1998, No. 2:186-191 [1035]

• Maiwald L. 1988. **Gripp-Heel®** (NL)/**Aconitum-Heel compositum** (B) in comparison with acetylsalicylic acid in treatment of influenza. In this study of 170 soldiers, the two medications were equally effective in treating influenza symptoms. *Biological Therapy* 1993, No. 1:2-8 [E 105]

6.1.3 In Vitro Studies

• Wagner H. 1986. Influencing phagocytosis activity of granulocytes with **Engystol® N**. In vitro test, single-blind study of mice. Rapid, marked increase in activity and increased resistance were observed after the first injection. *Biological Therapy* 1993, No. 1:43-49 [E 44 short version]

• Metelmann H, Glatthaar-Saalmüller R. 2000. Antiviral effect of **Euphorbium compositum S** Euphorbium compositum S has significant antiviral effects on respiratory syncytial virus and herpes simplex virus type 1 and minimal antiviral effects on influenza A. *Biomedical Therapy 2000*, No. 1:160-164 [E 121]

6.1.4 Drug Monitoring Studies

This section lists large-scale prospective studies, some of which involved more than 100 family practitioners or specialists and thousands of patients. This type of assessment is clearly more subjective than double- or single-blind studies, but the size of the population gives the data a relatively high degree of reliability after analysis, since any extreme assessments are moderated by the totality of the group. The large size of the population also means that even infrequently occurring adverse effects are almost certain to be detected. Finally, drug monitoring studies give a very clear picture of how commercially available medications are actually used, since the design of the study does not include guidelines and leaves the decision of how to administer the medication up to the attending physician. The most important studies conducted in the last few years are listed below.

• Frase W. 1995. **Luffa-Heel compositum** nasal spray and tablets in hay fever. Prospective study of 1,090 patients. Very good results were observed in 72 % of the patients treated. *Biological Therapy* 1995, No. 3:91-96 [1014]

• Weiser M. 1994. **Cerebrum compositum** in physiological disorders. Prospective study of 731 patients. Particularly effective in treating concussion, neurovegetative dystonia, and neurasthenia. *Biological Therapy* 1995, No. 3:85-90 [1012]

• Metelmann H. 1993. Intra-articular administration of **Zeel**® **P** in osteoarthritis of the knee. Prospective study involving 190 orthopedists, 1,845 patients, 16,974 injections. Marked improvement in symptoms was observed in 53 % of the patients and approximately 20 % were symptom-free after the course of therapy. *Biological Therapy* 1995, No. 1:12-20 [995]

• Zenner S. 1992. **Traumeel**® **S** ointment for musculoskeletal injuries. Prospective study involving 378 physicians, 3,422 patients. Best results observed in cases of hematoma, sprains, edema, and bursitis. *Biological Therapy* 1994, No. 3:204-211 [979]

• Metelmann H. 1992. **Euphorbium compositum-nasal spray S** in various types of rhinitis; 381 physicians, 3,510 patients. Best results were observed in acute rhinitis and sinusitis. *Biological Therapy* 1997, No. 3:.82-88 [977]

• Zenner S. 1992. Injection of **Traumeel**® **S** for musculoskeletal injuries. Prospective study of 3,241 patients. Best results observed in sprains, contusions, bursitis, and carpal tunnel syndrome. *Biological Therapy* 1994 No. 3:204-211 [974]

• Borho B. 1991.Treating vertigo with **Vertigoheel**®. Prospective study of 3 386 patients. Good to very good results were achieved in vertigo with unsteady gait, vertigo in elevators, and "everything-goes-black" episodes. *Biological Therapy* 1992, No. 3:281-288 [944]

In total, more than a thousand scientific studies (both articles and books) about Heel medications have been published worldwide and contain results of other prospective studies, empirical observations, reports of results in the field, etc.

Finally, it is fascinating to reflect that more than 300,000 injections of Heel medications are administered worldwide every day, not to mention all the tablets, drops, ointments, suppositories, sprays, gels, and single-dose vials that have been prescribed in the past 60 years and more. Indeed, Heel is a future with a tradition.

6.2 Conclusion

Heel laboratories conduct their scientific research in a professional manner and Heel medications and treatment strategies are scientifically well-founded. The lack of corroboration by experts from the allopathic sector says more about their own short-sightedness (which in the long run will be at the patient's expense) than about Heel's level of scientific research, which compares favorably with that of other, mainly allopathic, pharmaceutical laboratories in terms of GCP (Good Clinical Practice).

In scientific discussions, it is striking to note the extent of the ignorance of academics from the health care sector with regard to scientific studies on biological therapy. These professionals often fail to learn about the scientific basis of complementary therapies before developing critical opinions on the subject. Again, this violates the first rule of scientific inquiry, namely, the willingness to conduct unbiased investigation.

Volume 302 of the British Medical Journal (BMJ) (9 February 1991) contained a study by Kleijnen, Knipschild, and ter Riet analyzing the methods used internationally in the best scientific studies in alternative medicine. Not surprisingly, a Heel study (Zell, 1988; a double-blind study of Traumeel® S ointment versus placebo in sprains of the tarsal joint) topped the list. Although BMJ ranks as a standard reference in conventional medicine, most allopathic physicians have not read either this study or the metastudy on homeopathy by Linde in the September 1997 issue of the Lancet – surely also an allopathic reference.

Most physicians who work with Heel medications soon encounter more than adequate proof in daily practice and no longer feel the need for convincing scientific studies. Therefore, this chapter is directed to those who still doubt the scientific basis of Heel biotherapeutics in the hope that they will be able to abandon their bias and take the first safe steps into the fascinating world of complementary medicine.

The Scientific Basis of Antihomotoxic Therapy

7. References

(1)   Allendy. Les Nosodes. Annales Homéopathiques de l'Hospital St. Jacques, March/April 1932 (as quoted by Julian)

(2)   Bianchi I. Omotossicologia ed omeopatia classica ("Homotoxicology and Classical Homeopathy"). Revista Italiana di Omotossicologia 1985; 3 (2): 5–12

(3)   Bianchi I. Allopathie/Homotoxikologie/Klassische Homöopathie ("Allopathy/Homotoxicology/Classical Homeopathy"). ZDN „Dokumentation der besonderen Therapierichtungen und natürlichen Heilweisen in Europa". Vol. 1, no. 1, 1991; 560

(4)   Cahis M. Die Homöopathie experimentell bewiesen ("Experimental Proofs of Homeopathy"). Berliner Homöopathische Zeitschrift 1913; IV: 1–12

(5)   Danneberg G. Bacteriological and Virological Safety Assessment of Sinusitis Nosode. Battelle–Institut e.V., Final report 1991

(6)   Danner K. Übertragung spongiformer Enzephalopathien durch Arzneimittel – Grundzüge einer Risikobetrachtung ("Can Medications Transmit Spongiform Encephalopathy? An Outline of a Study of the Risks"). Pharm. Ind. 1991; 53 (7): 614–23

(7)   Das S. Ohne Inweltentgiftung keine ganzheitliche Therapie ("Without Detoxifying the Internal Milieu, No Holistic Therapy Succeeds"). Regensburg: Johannes Sonntag 1989; 44

(8)   Doutremepuich C. Ultra Low Doses. London, Washington D.C.: Taylor & Francis 1991

(9)   Fortier-Bernoville. Comment guerir par l'Homéopathie ("Healing Through Homeopathy") (as quoted by Julian)

(10) Frase W. Die Auto-Sanguis-Stufentherapie ("Graduated Auto-Sanguis Therapy"). Biol. Med. 1990; 19 (3): 152–8

(11) Gardes E. Effet d'une dilution infinitesimale d'Acide Nalixidique sur l'elimination de cette même molécule chez l'homme sain ("Effects of an Infinitesimal Dilution of Nalixidic Acid on Elimination of the Same Molecule in Healthy Humans"). Diplome Pharmacie 1988, Homéopathie française 1989; 77 (5): 60

(12) Gebhardt KH. Möglichkeiten und Grenzen der Homöopathie ("The Possibilities and Limits of Homeopathy"). Deutsche Apotheker Zeitung 1984; 124 (23): 1162

(13) Gedeon W. Empirische Heilmethoden in der Allgemeinmedizin ("Empirical Cures in General Medicine"). Heidelberg: Karl F. Haug 1986; 221

(14) Grabowski S. Die Grundlagen der Homotoxinlehre – Diagnostik und Therapie von Homotoxikosen ("The Fundamentals of the Homotoxin Theory – Diagnosis and Therapy of Homotoxicoses"). Berlin: undated.

(15) Gratz H. Erfahrungen mit Nosoden in der Kleintierpraxis ("Experience with Nosodes in the Small Animal Veterinary Practice"). Biol. Tiermed. 1987; 4: 14–7

(16) Heine H. Lehrbuch der biologischen Medizin ("Textbook of Biological Medicine"). Stuttgart: Hippokrates 1991; 104

(17) John J. Grundfragen zur antihomotoxischen Therapie ("Fundamental Questions about Antihomotoxic Therapy"). Biol. Med. 1977; 6 (5): 423–31

(18) Julian O. Materia medica der Nosoden ("Materia Medica of the Nosodes"). Heidelberg: Karl F. Haug 1983; 13

(19) Koch W.F. Das Überleben bei Krebs- und Viruskrankheiten ("Survival in Carcinomas and Viral Diseases"). Heidelberg: Karl F. Haug 1981

(20) Macleod G. A Veterinary Materia Medica and Clinical Repertory with a Materia Medica of the Nosodes. Saffron Walden: C.W. Daniel 1983; 167–80

(21) Mayr A, Büttner M. Paraspezifisches Immunsystem – Paraimmunisierung – Paraimmunität ("The Paraspecific Immune System – Paraimmunisation – Paraimmunity"). VET 1992; 7 (4): 31–7

(22) Metelmann H, Zenner S, Sonntag HG. Herstellung, Qualität und therapeutischer Einsatz von Nosodenpräparaten ("The Production, Quality, and Therapeutic Use of Nosode Preparations"). Biol. Med. 1988; 17: 217–24

(23) Mezger J. Gesichtete homöopathische Arzneimittellehre ("Selected Classification of Homeopathic Medications"). Fourth edition. Heidelberg: Karl F. Haug 1977; 1069

(24) Ordinatio Antihomotoxica et Materia Medica – Heel (as of 1 June 1989). Wissenschaftliche Abteilung der Biologische Heilmittel Heel GmbH, Baden-Baden

(25) Pischinger A. Das System der Grundregulation ("The Matrix Regulation System"). Eighth, revised edition. Heidelberg: Karl F. Haug 1990

(26) Reckeweg H.H. Homotoxine und Homotoxikosen. Grundlagen einer Synthese der Medizin ("Homotoxins and Homotoxicoses: The Fundamentals of a Synthesis in Medicine"). Second edition. Baden-Baden: Aurelia 1957

(27) Reckeweg H.H. Das Vikariationsphänomen zwischen Gesundheit und Siechtum ("The Phenomenon of Vicariation between Health and Illness"). Biol Med 1972; 1 (6): 121–37

(28) Reckeweg H.H. Homotoxikologie. Ganzheitsschau einer Synthese der Medizin ("Homotoxicology: A Holistic Review of a Synthesis in Medicine"). Sixth edition. Baden-Baden: Aurelia 1986

(29) Reckeweg H.H. Homoeopathia antihomotoxica. Eine gesichtete Arzneimittellehre ("Homoepathic Antihomotoxic Medications: Selected Classification of Homeopathic Medications"). Volume 1, fourth edition. Baden-Baden: Aurelia 1990

(30) Schmid F. Potenzierte Organotherapeutika. Wissenschaftliches Gutachten der Arzneimittelkommission für Biologische Medizin ("Potentized Organotherapeutics: A Scientific Deposition of the Medication Commission for Biological Medicine"). Karlsruhe 1991

(31) Sonntag H.G. Gutachten zur Unbedenklichkeit homöopathischer Nosoden-präparate ("Deposition on the Safety of Homeopathic Nosode Preparations"). Personal communication.1988 (Heidelberg University)

(32) Souza Magro I.A. et al. Redução da nefrotoxidade inducida por aminoglucosideos ("Use of Aminoglucosides to Reducing Induced Nephrotoxicity"). 41. Liga Medicorum Homoeopathicorum Internationalis Congress, Rio de Janeiro 1986

(33) Spitzy K.H. Arten der Arzneimittel ("Types of Medications"). ZDN „Dokumentation der besonderen Therapierichtungen und natürlichen Heilweisen in Europa". Vol.1, no.1, 1991; 562

(34) Stahl K.W. Wie kritisch sind Pharmakritiker? Zeel P, ein Testfall ("How Critical are Drug Critics? Zeel P: A Test Case"). Akt Rheumatol 1991; 16: 225–6

(35) Stock W, Metelmann H. Homöopathie – ein aktueller Beitrag zur biologischen Therapie ("Homeopathy: A Contribution of Topical Interest to Biological Therapy"). Reprinted from PTA 1985

(36) Straub O.C. Personal Communication, 1989 (Bundesforschungsanstalt für Viruskrankheiten der Tiere, Tübingen)

(37) Tobin S. A Holistic Viewpoint on Vaccinations – Schutzimpfungen aus ganzheitlich-medizinischer Sicht. In: Kongreßberichte des 3. Internationalen Kongresses für Veterinärhomöopathie der Int. Assoc. Vet. Hom. München: Müller & Steinicke 1992

(38) Virchow R. Künstliche und natürliche Therapie ("Artificial and Natural Therapy"). ZDN „Dokumentation der besonderen Therapierichtungen und natürlichen Heilweisen in Europa". Bd. 1, 1. Halbband 1991; 562

(39) Werthmann K. Therapeutischer Einsatz von Nosoden-Präparaten – Eine Anwendungsbeobachtung ("Therapeutic Use of Nosode Preparations: A Drug Monitoring Study"). Biol. Med. 1990; 19: 299–305

(40) ZDN „Dokumentation der besonderen Therapierichtungen und natürlichen Heilweisen in Europa ("Documentation of Specific Schools of Medical Theory and Natural Healing Methods in Europe"). Vol. 1, no. 1, 1991; 559